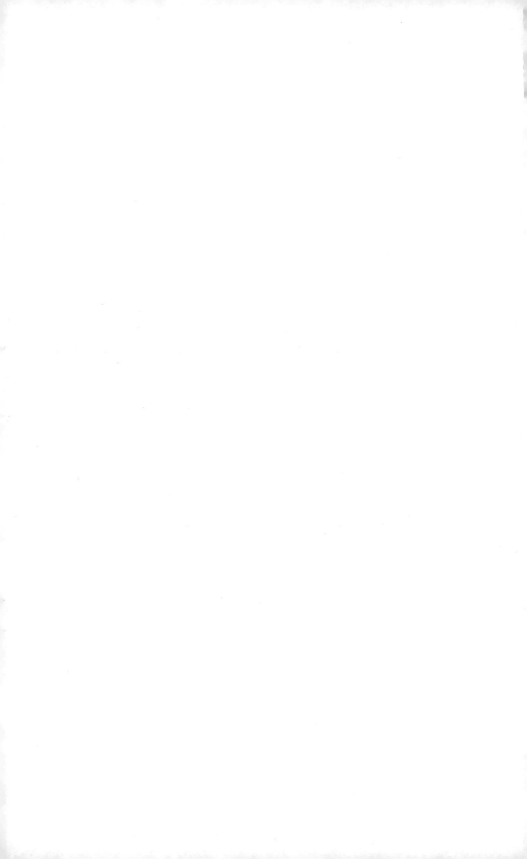

# RIPPED APART: LIVING MISDIAGNOSED

## WORKS BY DAVID BLACK

**Novels**
*Fast Shuffle*
*The Extinction Event*
*An Impossible Life*
*Peep Show*
*Minds*
*Like Father*

**Non-fiction**
*Medicine Man*
*Murder at the Met*
*The King of Fifth Avenue*
*Ekstasy*

**Plays**
*An Impossible Life*

**Poetry**
*Mirrors*

**Films**
*The Confession*
*Legacy of Lies*

**TV**
*Bluebloods*
*CopShop*
*CSI: Miami*
*The Bedford Diaries*
*The Education of Max Bickford*
*Sidney Lumet's 100 Centre Street*
*The Cosby Mysteries*
*EZ Streets*
*Law & Order*
*The Nasty Boys*
*H.E.L.P.*
*Gideon Oliver*
*Miami Vice*
*Hill Street Blues*

# RIPPED APART: LIVING MISDIAGNOSED

## Gary and Carol Stern's Epic Fight Against Malpractice in the American Health Care System

# DAVID BLACK

Skyhorse Publishing

Skyhorse Publishing books may be purchased in bulk at special discounts for sales promotion, corporate gifts, fund-raising, or educational purposes. Special editions can also be created to specifications. For details, contact the Special Sales Department, Skyhorse Publishing, 307 West 36th Street, 11th Floor, New York, NY 10018 or info@skyhorsepublishing.com.

Skyhorse® and Skyhorse Publishing® are registered trademarks of Skyhorse Publishing, Inc.®, a Delaware corporation.

Visit our website at www.skyhorsepublishing.com.

10 9 8 7 6 5 4 3 2 1

Library of Congress Cataloging-in-Publication Data is available on file.

Cover design by Kai Texel
Cover photo credit: Getty Images

Print ISBN: 978-1-5107-6265-7
Ebook ISBN: 978-1-5107-6766-9

Printed in the United States of America

Direct quotes are in quote marks. Indirect quotes are underlined.
All reportage from the trial is taken directly from the trial transcript and other publicly available court documents.
Some names have been changed.

For Gary

# Acknowledgments – from Carol Stern

I would like to thank Gary Stern, my husband, for showing me what unconditional love is.

Jeanette Bishop, my mom, for teaching me there is nothing you cannot accomplish so long as you love and trust in God and yourself and never take no for an answer.

Kenneth Laughlin, my son, for putting his life on hold more times than I can count.

Jade Laughlin, my granddaughter, for getting her Pop Pop (Gary) to smile when no one else could.

Kimberly Romero, my daughter, for all the moral support.

David and Stacey Stern, for always being there for Gary and me.

Donna Forehand, my niece. I was Gary's advocate and you were mine.

Miss Janet, Gary's home nurse, who was more of a family member than an employee.

Doctor Chun, for your love and understanding with Gary. I will always be indebted to you for the way you took care of my Gary.

Jay Miller, our attorney, for believing in us.

Linda and Rick Shade, my sister and brother-in-law, for your spiritual advice. God Bless you both.

Westview Baptist Church, for all the prayers and donations.

Mike Hagerty for believing in my story and introducing me to David Black.

David Black, the author, for helping me through the worst memories with love and compassion. I am happy to call you my friend.

The most important—GOD—for loving Gary and bringing his angels down to help me take care of him.

To everyone who helped me: thank you and I love you all.

God Bless,

Gary's Wife

# Acknowledgments – from Carol Stern

EARLY PRAISE FOR *RIPPED APART: LIVING MISDIAGNOSED*

"Crying. Devastating story, told with restraint. Has the inevitability of a Greek tragedy merged with the granular specificity of a law brief and a medical manual—yet somehow told as simply as possibly. Carol is a Greek heroine. You wisely step aside and let the story tell itself—though that's an illusion because stories don't tell themselves—you did. You make heroes out of regular suffering folk without hokum or schmaltz."
David Duchovny, actor and writer

"David Black is a genius."
Mort Gerberg, *New Yorker* cartoonist

"If you can only read one book before the world ends, this should be the one."
Richard Dreyfuss, actor and writer

"David Black is one of a very few writers who can tell a story of outrageous malfeasance without ever letting the outrage drown the plot. It's just one of the reasons I don't want his books to end."
John R. MacArthur, president and publisher of *Harper's Magazine*

"*Ripped Apart: Living Misdiagnosed* proves, once again, that David Black is one part sleuth and one part romantic, with a whole lot of style mixed in."
Tom Fontana, creator of the TV series *Oz* and many others; multiple Emmy winner.

PRAISE FOR DAVID BLACK'S PREVIOUS BOOKS

*FAST SHUFFLE*

"Black is a remarkable writer whose command of the hard-boiled and the sweet is matchless, not to mention his characters who embody both. Readers of this book are in for a wild ride from beginning to end with a lot of twists and turns that Black negotiates with elegance."
Carl Bernstein, Pulitzer Prize-winning journalist

*THE EXTINCTION EVENT*

"In a room full of tired thrillers and gumshoe capers, David Black's sensational new book is the life of the party. *The Extinction Event* sits at the table of Bradbury and *Chinatown*, Stieg Larsson and *CSI*."
Graydon Carter, journalist, author, and editor of *Vanity Fair*

"Hardboiled to perfection by a master of narrative alchemy. Here is a thriller yielding philosophical gold."
Frederic Morton, *New York Times* bestselling author of *A Nervous Splendor*

*LIKE FATHER: A NOVEL*

"Like Father is written with painful and beautiful understatement."
James Baldwin

"David Black's first novel is full of skill, humor, and humanity. The voice is individual, the dialogue real, the characters three-dimensional. The vision belongs to the great American tradition, but the eye that sees it is wholly original."
Anthony Burgess

"I loved it from the first paragraph. It's a rich, complex fascinating book; I ached for the characters and was sorry to say good-bye to them at the end."
Anne Tyler

*AN IMPOSSIBLE LIFE*

"Hilarious!"
Czeslaw Milosz, Noble Prize for Literature, 1980

"David Black's *An Impossible Life* is a brilliant depiction of a Jewish-American family unsparingly portrayed with all its craziness, eccentricity, and wild humor."
Erica Jong

# Table of Contents

---

# Trigger Warning

*Ripped Apart: Living Misdiagnosed* is a love story, a story about how love overcame the horror of a medical malpractice case—what Gary and Carol Stern went through.

It's *Romeo and Juliet* with the lovers separated not by a quarrel between two families, but by mortality.

The grimmer the ordeal that Gary went through, the more it testifies to Carol's love.

Gary spent three years with his internal organs on the outside of his body—but in addition to the medical misery and the successful landmark legal case, the book describes, through the lives of one couple, American health care at the street level, how health care affected an ordinary family. It describes in detail what it is like to suffer due to doctors' mistakes and their refusal to admit they made mistakes.

The gritty, sometimes gruesome, detail is important because (as in the movie MASH and the TV series *Nip/Tuck* and *The Knick,* and the Netflix show based on Dr. Liosa Sanders' popular column *Diagnosis,* and the *New York Times* paperback row-listed *Advice for Future Corpses and Those Who Love Them: A Practical Perspective on Death and Dying,* by Sallie Tisdale) the reality of what Gary and Carol Stern went through reflects what many people experience but are afraid to discuss: a silence that prevents others from revealing what they have experienced in American hospitals—in which 50 percent of the patients in hospitals are there due to being in a hospital; a silence that prevents the country from frankly dealing with the health-care crisis we face.

You can't understand what's going on in American health care without facing what happens in the operating room.

This is no polite narrative. As Gary said, euphemisms are lies. The book tells what suffering is like in all its honest detail and how American health care fails.

We read about people going through suffering because it gives us the ability to deal with our own suffering.

If you are squeamish, stop reading. If you want the truth about what goes on in the human heart, turn the page.

There has never been a more honest book written about the dark side of American health care—and about love that knows no boundaries, not even death.

*Between grief and nothing I will take grief.*

William Faulkner, *The Wild Palms*

# Part One

---

For I know the plans I have for you...
to give you a future and a hope.

Jeremiah 29:11

# 1

Carol Stern realized her husband Gary was sick in May of 2011, when she came into the living room of their townhouse in Baltimore and found him sitting on the edge of the couch, rocking back and forth. *The Three Stooges* was on TV. His favorite. He identified with all of them, each for a different reason. He talked most about Mo; but, if he had to choose the Stooge he figured he was like, he'd pick Curly. The smart one. Carol used to tell him, "Do you realize how much violence is going on in there?" He'd say, "But it's funny. Okay?"

Gary knew about violence. He and his brother, David, were bail bonds-men and bounty hunters. Not so funny. Jewish bounty hunters. Okay, a *little* funny.

Carol would shrug and say, "Go ahead and watch it."

Gary was always watching "The Stooges." Either that or a cooking show or QVC. He loved to order things, often electronic equipment, or shoes, or ties. Two of each. But mostly he ordered jewelry for Carol. He never bought just one of anything, either. Even later, when they were together, Gary couldn't buy just one Boston terrier. (To get two, he had to take three: Butchy, Zenny, and Princie.)

Gary didn't like just one of anything.

"Except," Carol would say, "his wife. He wanted only one wife."

Even at the end, after the doctors misdiagnosed him and gutted him and his intestines were open to the world for almost three years, after the suffering and anger and laughter and despair, after the fights with the government (including the White House) over health care and the law suits, it was, Carol thought, ironic that Gary had two funerals: one Jewish funeral in Baltimore at Sol Levinson Funeral Home with Cantor Tom King from Beth El Synagogue for Gary's family, and one Christian funeral in Martinsburg, West Virginia, with Pastor Bryan Dugger at Westview Baptist, Carol's mother's church, for Carol's family.

The congregation in Martinsburg had sent money when Carol and Gary were destitute and having trouble paying Gary's medical bills. They also had sent a prayer quilt to Gary, which members of the congregation had made.

Carol didn't realize how many people cared about them. She corrected herself: how many people cared about Gary.

For Carol, it was always about Gary.

Even after Carol and Gary told his family that they were in love and intended to get married, his family hadn't visited with Carol much. Gary's sister Barbara didn't know Gary was dating anyone, so hearing about Carol was a surprise.

"When I first met Carol," Barbara said, "Wow, she has the same color hair as mom's,"

They were at a family dinner, which Barbara thought was a little uncomfortable. It was obvious that Gary and Carol were in love, surprising, because Gary and Carol had such opposite personalities. Gary was introverted, Carol extroverted. Barbara figured their relationship was just a fling.

Carol struck Stacey, David's wife, as down-to-earth, no nonsense, grounded. She was recovering from her terrible second marriage, and Stacey could tell Carol was emotionally fragile. Stacey liked how much in love Gary was. And how much Gary was taking care of her.

"He did everything for her," Stacey said. "One hundred percent."

# 2

That first day when Gary got sick, he dismissed the pain. When he was younger—as a child and in 2000—he'd had Crohn's Disease, inflammation of the gastrointestinal tract, which can occur anywhere from the mouth, the esophagus, down to the anus.

Gary figured that's what was causing him pain.

"Don't call 911 or anyone," Gary said. "I'll take some aspirin. I'll be okay."

But Gary wasn't okay. All week the pain got worse. Finally, Carol went into the bathroom, closed the door, and called for help. When EMS arrived, Gary was furious. He could handle the pain, he told Carol.

"Just let them check you out," Carol said.

EMS thought Gary was having a heart attack, because his blood pressure was so high. They put him into the ambulance and took him to Sinai Hospital. Carol tried to follow behind in their white van. She didn't know where the hospital was and, trying not to lose the ambulance, she got a camera ticket for running a red light. Of course, she'd run a red light. She didn't want to lose Gary.

# 3

Carol and Gary met in 2002 at the Cancun Cantina, a huge club at 7501 Old Telegraph Road, in Hanover, Maryland, where Carol went regularly and that Gary had recently found. In the front room, geezers, who had left their walkers by the sidelines, and toddlers in jeans and Western snap-button shirts joined the young men and women in their twenties and older couples in their thirties and forties and fifties in line dances. Colored lights bathed the people on the dance floor red and the guys and gals gathered three deep at the bar in blue.

Carol was on the dance floor. Red.

Gary was standing at the bar. Blue.

Four months after Carol had moved to Baltimore for her job, someone reminded her about the Cantina. Years earlier, when she was on the road, on one of her rare nights off, she had wandered into the Cantina. From the highway, you couldn't miss the huge neon sign out front. It was a mild summer night. She had parked her car and sat for a while with the window open, smoking a cigarette and casing the place. There were two dozen Harleys in the parking lot, which could be a good or bad sign. Depending. Men in cowboy hats and cowboy boots and beautiful women streamed into the club. Everyone looked happy. All the men were tipping their hats to each other and holding the door open for their dates. Carol got out of her car and went inside, past the life-sized Captain Morgan in the entrance hallway.

She smelled the leather from the boots, the different types of perfume and cologne. There was lots of laughter. Carol could feel the pounding of the dancing cowboys and cowgirls on the hardwood floor.

Carol had just gotten out of a horrific relationship and had forgotten about the good things in life. It had been more than fourteen years since she had been anywhere like the Cantina.

In five minutes, she was on the floor line-dancing. She couldn't believe she still remembered the moves. After thirty-five minutes, she hit the bar—where she met her first dance partner, Richard, who—when she moved back to the area—became a close friend. Richard was a hard-core biker. He owned a few boats for crabbing. The rest of the time, he drank and danced and drank some more. Richard loved the Cantina, and everyone at the Cantina loved him. He became Carol's protector.

"Not that I needed protection," Carol said.

She could take care of herself.

Carol explained, "The Cantina was about everyone looking out for each other."

In the huge back room—a separate bar for rock-and-roll—most of the dancers were all the same age. Twenties or twenties-wanna-be's. Unlike the Western bar, this room smelled of sour beer and human sweat.

Carol rarely went into that room.

After she had moved to Baltimore and became a Cantina regular, Carol met another close friend, Sindie Moluski, who had long blond hair and high cheekbones. On the dance floor, Sindie was beautiful to watch. Carol joined the dancers, danced for a half hour, and went to the bar to get a drink. Sindie came up to her and said <u>she</u> was beautiful to watch. Carol? Beautiful to watch? Carol thought Sindie couldn't be matched. Carol couldn't believe what Sindie was saying: This woman who looked as if she were dancing on air was saying Carol was a great dancer.

They became best friends. Everyone at the Cantina knew them and wanted to learn from them. While they were on the dance floor, no one sat on Carol's and Sindie's bar stools. If someone didn't know the drill, the bartender made sure their bar stools were empty and waiting for them. Sindie and Carol never understood why. They weren't often at the bar.

Carol went to the Cantina every Friday and Saturday night and often on Wednesday, Ladies Night. Carol and Sindie were Cantina trend-setters.

Whenever they wore an outfit, within two or three weeks they'd see the same outfit on a half dozen other women.

Sindie—a single mother of two—worked for Verizon in computer management and was going to an online college, getting two master's degrees. She was about Carol's size: five feet five inches tall, 125 pounds, blond hair, brown eyes. She was eight years younger than Carol. Everyone assumed they were sisters. Their friend Lori, another blond about Carol's and Sindie's size —everyone at the Cantina called them The Three Blonds—hung out with them, but didn't do a lot of dancing. She preferred sitting at the bar, meeting and talking to people.

One night, The Three Blonds were sitting at the bar, watching everyone dance. Four men from the Rock-and-Roll side passed them. One of the guys rubbed his privates against Carol's knee. Four times in a row. Carol punched him in the stomach hard enough that he threw up. Within seconds, security was there. The four Rock-and-Rollers got banned from the Cantina. The Three Blonds laughed about the incident. All they had to do was look at the bartender a certain way and security or one of their friends would be right there. They were safe at the Cantina.

Another night, when Carol went to the ladies' room, three women were talking about "a blonde stuck-up bitch." They meant Sindie. Carol told them they had no idea what they were talking about. Carol took the one who was talking trash about Sindie to the bar where Sindie was sitting. Within ten minutes, Sindie was on the dance floor teaching the Trash Talker the Texas stomp. After that, anytime the three catty women came back to the Cantina they always came up to the Three Blonds to say hello and give them hugs.

Yet another night—in her usual cowboy boots, jeans, cowboy shirt, and cowboy hat, all black like a female Johnny Cash, Carol was taking a break from teaching dances and was high-stepping around the floor, dancing just for the joy of it. Gary—not in Western gear—watched her. She watched him watching her.

> Remember when I was young and so were you
> And time stood still and love was all we knew

Alan Jackson's "Remember When," which was playing, became their song.

We lived and learned, life threw curves
There was joy, there was hurt
Remember when

Carol knew a mutual friend had encouraged Gary to come to the Cantina that night to meet her. And Carol knew Gary knew. And Gary knew Carol knew he knew.

"I was cocky back then," Carol said.

For a couple weeks, Gary watched her teaching people. She talked to everybody. Helped others have fun. Gary liked that.

Carol was by the bar. Gary was on an upper level along one wall. When Carol saw him, she gestured for him to come over.

"He had the nerve to shake his head no at me," Carol said.

And he gestured for her to go over to him.

Carol shook her head no.

A stand-off.

Gary pointed to the stairs halfway between.

"That's all it took," Carol said. "He wasn't bowing to me. I wasn't bowing to him. From that point on, it was 50/50."

Together and equal.

"Oh, goodness," Carol said, "that's how it started."

Gary wore a thick, gold bracelet, which he put on Carol.

When Carol handed it back to Gary, he said, "It looks better on you."

"Yeah," Carol said, "but it's yours."

The bracelet became a running joke—until it stopped being a joke and became a commitment.

"Doesn't the music make you want to dance?" Carol asked him.

Gary said he didn't know how.

He did know how. Before Gary met Carol, he'd danced at the bar he and David owned. But, for some reason, Carol intimidated him. Maybe it was the all-black outfit. And because Carol was the best dancer at the Cantina.

"I'll get you dancing." Carol led him by the hand onto the floor—where she, in fact, got him dancing.

"About ten, fifteen years ago," Gary later said, "line dancing, country dancing . . . there were a lot of places to go . . . [I]t wasn't about drinking and partying, it was about everybody just in a big group having a good time."

A shared communal interest.

"She started to teach me, help me," Gary said.

He arranged to meet her later by the hot dog stand. "She thought I meant the one right outside the bar, but it was the one across the street." At the 7/11. Gary waited until 2:30 a.m. Carol—at the other hotdog stand—waited until 4. They each thought the other stood them up.

"So," Carol said, "we lost touch."

Carol went on a sabbatical—actually a working vacation—to the Dallas-Fort Worth area, for three weeks.

Gary told a friend, "I'm giving her one more week."

But three weeks later, he showed up on a Wednesday night, which was ladies night. Carol was back—in her cowboy boots and hat, a little dressier than usual, more make-up than usual, her long blond hair loose. All the guys wanted to dance with her and with Sindie.

But Carol wanted to dance only with Gary.

Gary was gallant. When they walked outside, he made sure he was next to the street and Carol was on the inside. Carol was charmed.

They had only dated a few times when, one Friday night, Carol got sick. Either she drank too much or the drinks didn't mix well with some medication. She hung about the sidelines, not dancing, knocking back shots called Blow Jobs, whiskey and whipped cream. After last call, Gary followed Carol into the parking lot. Gary lived in one direction from the Cantina in Owings Mills; Carol lived in the opposite direction, in Laurel. Gary said he was going to follow her home to make sure she made it safely. She didn't. Four blocks from her apartment, she pulled to the side of the road and vomited all over her car and all over her black jump-suit.

When Gary opened her door, the stench from the vomit hit him in the face. It didn't bother him. Nothing about Carol ever bothered Gary. Carol, her black cowboy hat askew, beamed up blearily at Gary. After Gary determined that Carol was okay, he started laughing. He helped her out of her Grand Am and put her in his Corvette, which he drove to her building. He led her to her second floor apartment. Carol was so out of it, the next morning she had no memory of going home and taking a shower—which she did. She did remember waking up with wet hair in fresh-smelling clothes. Her roommates gathered around and told her that her boyfriend was awesome. He had cleaned her up.

Gary interrupted them, bringing in coffee, eggs, and orange juice. And Carol's car keys. After dropping off Carol at her apartment and cleaning her up and tucking her into bed, he had gotten a bucket, soapy water, and sponges and had driven back to Carol's car, which he cleaned.

# 4

Gary and Carol took it slow.

"It was my first marriage," Gary said. "I was in no rush. I wanted to marry. But I wanted to marry once, and she was it."

Gary would woo Carol for five years until on May 1, 2006, they got married. They both took their vows seriously. They wanted to be ready—to be sure. Once they were man and wife, when they weren't working they were always together.

Gary had a tendency to cut himself down. Despite his success at sports and his young Al Pacino good looks, he was insecure. Maybe because he—like Pacino—was short, the result of medication he'd had to take when he was a kid.

When he was around thirteen, Gary had a severe case of diarrhea and cramping in his stomach. Gary was scared. Sonny and Peggy, Gary's parents, took him to a doctor, who sent him to various specialists, who diagnosed it as some kind of inflammation. Probably Crohn's Disease. Back then not a lot was known about Crohn's Disease.

Gary took Prednisone, a steroid, and Azulfidine, used to treat ulcerative colitis and Crohn's Disease, both of which helped, but which had bad side effects. Gary stopped growing.

"Adolescence, puberty," Gary said, "the medication cut it all off."

The Prednisone blew Gary up and made him look (Gary thought) like a balloon animal.

Because the illness stunted his growth, Gary became introverted and angry.

He was five feet six. Carol was five feet.

She loved short men.

Carol could tell that the women in his past hadn't treated him right. Carol determined to build up his confidence, to make sure Gary knew he was as wonderful on the inside as he was on the outside. She encouraged one of her girlfriends at the Cantina to kiss him. On the cheek. Finally, she told him, "Gary, you were afraid to come up to me because all the other men were coming up to me. Do you really think that I would be with somebody that wasn't worthy?"

For their first Halloween together (in 2003), Carol dressed Gary up as a sheik. She and some of her friends dressed up as his harem girls. A confidence builder. It wasn't long before, when they danced, they had the whole floor to themselves. Gary liked to finish each dance by dipping Carol. When Gary entered the Cantina, the DJ stopped whatever song was on to announce, "Hey, everybody, get ready. Gary's in the house," and would play "Remember When." Everybody would applaud.

It took a year for Gary to stop putting himself down. By then, despite his initial shyness, Gary became popular at the Cantina. And he became more confident with Carol. That December, he arranged a surprise birthday party for Carol at a restaurant in Columbia, Maryland, which in 2016 *Money* magazine listed as the best place to live in America. His present to Carol was a diamond bracelet, a second bracelet to match the gold bracelet he had put on Carol's wrist when they first met. They were the first diamonds Carol had ever owned. She still wears the bracelet.

## 5

Born on September 7, 1963, Gary was the third of four children. Barbara—Barbara Lee Clabaugh—was the first born, Steven Mark (who everyone called Stevie) was second. Then came Gary and David, who were born only thirteen months apart. (David in October 1964). They felt like twins. Carol claimed they looked like twins. At Fort Garrison Elementary School, Gary was held back a year, so Gary and David ended up in the same class. They had the same friends.

"We did everything together," David said.

In everything they did, from basketball to the racehorses, Gary's family was competitive, but Gary was the best in everything. From childhood, Gary was a great athlete—which would come in handy when he and David opened the bar in Baltimore and they had to give rowdies the bum's rush. When they opened their bail bond office, they became their own bounty hunters, tracking down and bringing in bail jumpers. And, later, Gary needed the strength to survive the physical traumas of both his illness and his treatments.

Middle and high schools were in Pikesville. For college, they both went to Towson for two years, which was enough time to prove that Gary and David weren't cut out for college. Sonny, their dad, got David a job with a friend of his, Michael Lasky, who owned a sports consulting company, Mike Warren Sports. Gamblers called in and paid for advice on where to place their bets. David was making good money.

With money from his parents, Gary bought a bar, The Twilight in Marley Park, Glenn Burnie, Maryland, 648 Annapolis Boulevard, a tough neighborhood. The bar was run down, like the people who went there. There was live music on weekends, lots of drugs, lots of fights. When David and Stacey would drop by, the bikers who hung out there tried to kiss Stacey. The bar needed some serious muscle. Sonny knew a couple of criminals in the neighborhood. They could fight, and they could cook. And one of them knew how to run a business. Sonny figured the guy would be a good manager. After about two years, Gary's partner set the bar up to get robbed by one of his pals, who slept in the back room, where Gary and Sonny found him passed out with stolen liquor and cash, a couple of thousand dollars, the night's take, as well as some liquor. Gary fired him.

Gary wanted David to be his new partner. For a while, David tried to do both jobs—the sports betting and the bar—at the same time. David soon decided he had to quit Mike's business, which he did.

They sank $100k into gutting and remodeling the bar. Gary and David did most of the work. They added a real restaurant. They mopped floors, ran the bar and the kitchen, and knocked troublemakers upside the head for a profitable eight years. Occasionally family members—like Gary and David's sister Barbara—pitched in. They changed the name to Doc's Restaurant and Lounge. <u>Doc</u> was a nickname Sonny gave Gary when Gary was a kid and volunteered at a hospital. The bar T-shirt showed a doctor with a Snidely Whiplash upturned mustache, stethoscope around his neck, physician's mirror strapped to his forehead, tongue depressors in his white tunic's breast pocket, holding a house-call bag in his left hand and a beer in his right.

At the pre-opening party, there was a brawl in the parking lot between Doc's bartender, his friends, and a bunch of customers. After that, they arranged for bikers to be the bar's bouncers. A local, Jimmy, got stone drunk and started mouthing off. Al, one of the Biker Bouncers, picked the guy up by his neck and walked him outside. Jimmy's friends pulled knives on the biker, who was ready to fight, but the Knife Boys backed off.

Gary and David didn't see much sunlight. They opened at 6:00 in the morning and closed at 2:00 the next morning. Factory workers from the Curtis Bay area, an industrialized waterfront, stopped in on their way to and from their shifts in the factories.

"This guy, Tim, came in during the day," David said, "and was sitting at a high top. He ordered a Budweiser. I looked over, and he was snorting lines [of coke] on the table. I said, 'Tim you can't do that in here.' He snorted the last line, chugged the beer, and said 'I'm leaving.'"

By then, no one wanted to face the Biker Bouncers.

Two coke dealers who lived in the neighborhood helped protect the bar. In exchange, Gary and David ignored their dealing to the customers.

One of the dealers spent thousands of dollars in the draw poker machine. One night, he lost $2,000. He put his fist through the machine's glass and then threw it to the ground.

Another night, Gary and David returned to the bar and found two guys hanging around. Both were stone drunk. David knew something was up.

Gary and David half-owned the bar's Poker machine, and split the profits with a guy named Ray who regularly came by and rolled the quarters, as he did that night.

Ray glanced at the machine and said, "Dave, Gary, this isn't my lock." They cut the lock. The machine was empty.

Gary and David went outside and checked the pick-up truck owned by the two guys who had been hanging around. On the floor was a pile of quarters. They called the police, who helped Gary and David get their quarters back. Gary and David barred the two guys who stole from the poker machine for a month.

The bar worked great for a year or so. The remodeling was good for the neighborhood. But the cops came and said Anne Arundel County was banning the poker machines.

You can remove them, the cops said, or we'll do it for you in a couple of weeks.

The poker machines represented a big part of their profits, which were affected because the bar kept getting skimmed or robbed often by regulars. The whole scene was getting crazier and crazier. Everyone was sleeping with everyone except David, who was with Stacey. Gary was screwing the barmaids and the girls who came in.

There were bar fights every night. On more than one occasion, one of the female patrons reached over and pulled the barmaid's hair out of her head.

Another night, a guy—six foot four, 220 pounds, probably on PCP—ripped the urinal off the bathroom wall, went outside, and threw it through a car window. Six cops clubbed him. He didn't feel a thing.

And termites were eating the bar away.

In 1989, when the novelty of the new bar wore off and fewer customers were showing up, they sold the bar to the cop who had helped them get their quarters back.

"We fabricated a few things to make the bar look a little better than it really was," David admitted.

For Gary and David, it was time for a change.

# 6

Gary and David's older brother, Stevie, was in law school and working in Sonny's office. Sonny knew a bail-bondsman—Fred Frank—who used to come over to play in Sonny's regular Sunday basketball games. Fred owned Fred Frank Bail Bonds, one of the biggest operations in Maryland. Fred put Stevie in touch with one of his employees. Together they opened up Courtside Bail Bonds. For 10 percent of the amount of a bail, they would pledge the full amount.

Sonny steered Courtside's first client to the Courtside. For a $250,000 bail, they got a $25,000 fee. Not bad, David thought, for Courtside's first bail. Their second client—also recommended by Sonny—was for $250,000 bail, which meant Courtside collected another $25,000 fee.

"Bam Bam," David said, "I want to do this."

Gary, David, and Barbara all went to school and got their bail bonds licenses—another 24/7 business.

Stevie and his partner were fighting over money, so they split up. Sonny decided Gary, David, and Stevie should go into business together. They called it Brothers Bail Bonds. It's been called Brothers Bail Bonds since 1989.

"Our professional bail bond staff will spring into action to help you understand the bail process and make this difficult situation as easy as possible for you," one of their ads said. "Whether you are in jail for a traffic ticket, warrant, DUI, or any other type of violation, we understand what you are going through."

"If you want to see your mother, call Brothers," was their motto. They even filmed a TV commercial.

When criminals wouldn't show up for court, Gary, David, and Stevie had to go after them so Brothers Bail Bonds wouldn't be on the hook for the full amount of the bail. Gary and David depended on Stevie, who was older, to take the lead. One time, David and Stevie went to pick up a young man for FTA—Failing To Appear in court.

"The guy was arrested for beating a friend with a pipe," David said. "We tracked him down and locked him up, no problem."

Not long after Brothers Bail Bonds opened, on December 1, 1990, Stevie overdosed. Thirty years old. In high school, Stevie had taken Quaaludes, but his drug of choice became cocaine—although he stole a bottle of Methadone from a clinic. He didn't know how to use it and drank too much. He may have had other drugs in his system at the time. The next day, Sonny and Peggy found him on the floor. Dead.

Running Brothers Bail Bonds without Stevie meant Gary and David went after the FTAs: mostly surveillance, mostly dull, waiting and watching. But after the waiting and watching, they kicked open doors. Pumped on adrenalin, reckless, and scared shitless, Gary was always the first one through the door.

"Gary was an awesome person," Kelly, an old friend, once said. "He was a badass."

Gary and David could go through peoples' homes, because they had warrants.

"We can go through the house as much as we want," David said, "as long as it is the address the defendant gave to the courts or, if we have a suspicion he is in another house, we can ask the police to make them let us in."

Most of the time the homes were unlocked. Gary and David would walk right in, guns drawn. Once they burst into an apartment, where the guy they were after was writing something down, ignoring the baby roaches crawling over his hand.

"We went to arrest a client named Donald," David said. "He was an addict, who lived in a neighborhood that was a cesspool for drugs and everything else. We walked right in the front door, past the grandfather sleeping on a rocking chair, and up the steps to meet Donald. Gary and I had guns drawn, and Donald had his back to us."

Donald was six-five, 280 pounds. His shoulders were wider than Gary and David standing side-by-side.

"Donald," David said, "we need to go."

Donald turned around, smoking a crack pipe, and said about Gary's and David's guns, Dave, you don't need that.

David was shaking, saying to himself, "Yes, I do."

If Donald didn't comply, David didn't know what would happen. Gary never backed down. But Donald let himself be led away. Gary and David delivered him to the court.

A drug dealer named Alan Pocock, a repeat offender, was giving Gary and David a lot of business. He ended up going away for ten years. In jail, no bail. That affected their bottom line.

Any story that begins with a one-armed Mexican is a good story.

The Mexican—Miguel Cesar, a con man—could drive a car and text and salt a sandwich at the same time," David said. "He could do five different things at once."

Gary and David bailed him out—a $40,000 bond. Cesar was a no-show in court. Gary and David went looking for him, starting with his family, who claimed they had no idea where Cesar was. Gary and David rummaged through their house at all hours of the night to disrupt their lives until—Gary and David hoped—the family would tell them where Cesar was. They never did.

For months, Gary and David investigated. No luck. They paid the court the whole $40k bond. The clock started ticking. They had ten years to deliver Cesar to the court, which then would give them their $40k back. They questioned Cesar's friends and enemies. They advertised on a show called *Maryland's Most Wanted*, which covered fugitives.

There was a big Mexican population in Fells Point, a section of Baltimore. One night, Gary got a call from someone in the area saying he knew where Cesar was. Cesar owed the guy money. Since the guy couldn't collect from Cesar, he figured he'd rat him out for the reward Gary and David were offering.

Gary and David met the guy at their father's, Sonny's, downtown office. The guy drew them a map of Monterey, Mexico, where Cesar was hiding out with his parents. Gary and David contacted the Federales in Monterey, who spotted Cesar. The Federales told Gary and David they would push Cesar over the border for $10,000.

"Ten k," David said. "We crapped our pants."

But $40k minus $10k still left Gary and David $30,000. They contacted the Maryland State's Attorney, and said they'd get Cesar over the border into Laredo, Texas. They wanted Maryland to help them extradite him. The State's Attorney said they would not help. Gary and David filed a petition: if the state wouldn't help, the court had to release Brothers from the obligation of the bail and return their money.

The district court judge denied the motion, saying that unless Cesar was in Baltimore, there was nothing the court could do.

"Judge," David said, "you're missing the point."

Either they needed help getting Cesar back to Maryland or, if the state wouldn't help, they needed relief.

The judge gave David the once-over and denied their motion.

"We appealed it," David said. "It went to the circuit court, which ruled in our favor."

They got the whole $40k from the court without having to bring Cesar back from Mexico.

Even when they were doing dull surveillance work, "it was great," David said, "just hanging with my brother."

They didn't write bonds on prostitutes, "because," Carol said, "they never show up."

David agreed.

"Women pros," he said, "go from city to city. And, even if they get arrested somewhere else, we don't know about it. It's easy for them to run."

On a few occasions, they had to get a death certificate so they could get their money back from the court.

They bailed out a guy named Edward Clyde, who stabbed a good friend of his and left him for dead. The friend did not die, and Clyde did not show up for his court date. Gary and David contacted his girlfriend Sue, who had co-signed the agreement with Brothers. She was responsible for Clyde showing up in court. If he skipped, she would owe the amount of the bail: $35k. She refused to pay. Gary and David followed her around during the day and went through "her shithole of a house" at all times of the night. They knew she was hiding Clyde. One night, they got a call from the FBI, who she had called, complaining about Gary and David. Gary wasn't sure he believed the call was authentic. He called the local FBI office and got the guy who had called them. They explained what was going on. He helped them by getting a no-flight warrant on Clyde. For months, Gary and David followed Sue without luck. On Memorial Day weekend, Gary and David were working at Sonny's office when they got a call.

"Are you looking for Edward Clyde?" the caller asked. "He's at Coco's Pub on Hartford Road."

"What do you want out of this?" Gary asked.

"Nothing," the caller said. "I just want him locked up."

"Why?"

The caller didn't say.

Gary and David drove to Coco's Pub.

David walked through the place and did not see Clyde. David went in, as Gary was hot headed and might throw an unnecessary punch. David went back to the car, where he and Gary sat for an hour or so, waiting for Clyde to come out. They got hungry. Together, they went into Coco's to get some fried chicken, which they ate back in the car.

David went through the bar again, and again he did not see Clyde. On his way back through the parking lot to the stake-out car, David saw Mary— Clyde's girlfriend (who owed them $35,000) tooling down the street in what David called "her piece of shit green SUV" with a guy in the passenger seat. It was Clyde, who she dropped off at a house.

"We had him," David said.

To make sure they kept him, they called one of their employees— Andy Bettencourt—who helped them with bail-jumpers they thought would be risky, someone who might retaliate. Gary and David had bailed out Bettencourt a number of times on drug charges. No fool, Bettencourt clocked how much money Gary and David were making and asked how he could get into the business. He took the necessary courses and got his license and Gary and David hired him. Bettencourt was black and could bring in clients Gary and David might not be able to reach. He wrote bails in the middle of the night when Gary and David didn't want to run down to the courts.

Bettencourt was six-five, 210 pounds. Scary.

One day, Gary and David were trying to kick down a hotel door. Unsuccessfully.

"Get your size fourteens over here," Gary said.

Inside the room, Gary and David cuffed the fugitive. While walking him to their car, Bettencourt punched the guy in the jaw.

That, Bettencourt said, is for making us chase you around town.

Another time, Bettencourt watched the back door of a bail-jumper as Gary and David knocked on the front door. The jumper opened the door. They barged in and handcuffed him. No problem. They took him to the city jail, lucky to avoid violence once more.

Gary and David bailed out an acquaintance of David's, Malcome Yeats, for $7,500 for a domestic violence beef with his wife. Yeats called from the court saying, "David, they want to give me six months in jail. I'm not going to jail."

David said, "You wanna bet?"

Yeats decided to just walk out of the courthouse.

Gary and David asked a mutual friend where Yeats was staying. The friend told them. Gary and David called the police for back-up, because Yeats was six-two, 250 pounds. Another Donald.

"We wanted to be sure there were going to be no problems," David said.

When Yeats was first arrested, he had threatened cops in the police station, so, when Gary mentioned Yeats's name, the cops sent the cavalry. Gary and David walked up the street with ten officers, all with shotguns and sidearms drawn. The police wanted Yeats worse than Gary and David did.

At Yeats's house, Gary went with five officers to the back door while David went with five to the front door. At both doors, they were backed up by K-9 units. Above them hovered a police helicopter.

Yeats let his dogs out the back door. Gary, the five cops, and the K-9 unit had to run for their lives, jumping over a fence, where one cop split his pants. Yeats's dogs were known for being especially fierce.

Yeats walked out the front door and asked David, "What's up?"

Once he was cuffed, the cops wanted to mace him. A bad idea.

Three fugitives that Gary and David arrested were naked when the brothers burst into their homes. One, a female, was in the attic, also naked. David, the married brother, told Gary, "You are going up to get her."

They tracked another naked guy, who was snorting cocaine and having sex with his girlfriend. Without dismounting, he asked, Can we do this tomorrow?

At the third fugitive's house Gary and David had to kick in the door. The place had no furniture. In the upstairs bedroom, they found a topless woman, just sitting on the floor.

"Where the fuck is he," David asked about the fugitive.

I don't know, she said.

"Put some clothes on," Gary said.

She did, and then ratted out her boyfriend.

Over almost thirty years, Gary and David arrested between one hundred and one hundred and fifty bail-jumpers.

They each carried a Glock 19.

"The sucker was heavy," Carol said.

Carol still has the handcuffs and leg chains Gary used.

# 7

In between dances at the Cantina, Carol told Gary her story.

Carol was born on December 16, 1960, in a Catholic hospital in Enid, Oklahoma.

"I was delivered to my mom in a Christmas stocking," Carol said.

She had three older sisters from her mom's—Jeanette's—previous marriage. They were named Linda, Marcia, and Karen, and Carol never considered them half-sisters.

"We were all sisters," Carol said.

Carol, whose father was Catholic, was raised Catholic.

"Nuns rapping my knuckles," she said. "The whole business."

Carol joined the Baptist Church— like her grandmother, who had been raised Catholic and became a Baptist.

"She got dipped," Gary said. Baptized.

Carol's maternal grandmother came from Moultrie, Georgia. She died when Carol's mother was a year and a half old.

"You're going to think I'm crazy," Carol said, "but I knew her mom"—Carol's grandmother—"because she used to come to me."

Carol's grandmother had long hair and appeared in a long white dress. Carol could see through her "just barely."

"She came to me several times," Carol said.

Carol first encountered this mysterious presence in the middle of June, 1965, when she was four-and-a-half years old: her earliest memory.

"We lived in military housing," Carol said. "The houses were more like town homes with four families living in each building. There was a play area in the back with a basketball court. It was a Sunday morning. I remember this because I took my mom the Sunday paper so she could read me the comics."

Jeanette's bedroom was on the third floor. The window over the bed was open. Carol's brother, a baby, was waking up from his morning nap.

"He was crying," Carol said. "My mom told me she would be right back. I was lying in her bed, and I could hear the kids play in the back. I stood on my mom's bed to watch them. I must of been watching them for a while because I decided to sit on the window sill. The screen gave way. Everything went so slow. A woman was holding me in her arms as I was falling down like I was a feather. I could see the kids running to me as if they were going to catch me. The next thing I remember was having a cast on my left leg."

Because Carol's dad was in the military, they moved around a lot, finally landing in San Diego in 1966.

They moved to Gateway military housing, about forty minutes away from the Marine Corps Air Station and the Miramar Naval Air Station. In military housing. Carol's father, Kenneth Elmer Bishop, adopted Linda, Marcia, and Karen.

From 1954 to 1960, Kenneth was in the Air Force, a skillful enough flight instructor to train The Blue Angels.

"We would fly across country," Carol said. "I always felt safe with my dad flying, that's why I love to fly so much."

In 1962, Kenneth joined the Navy. Carol's father gave students flying lessons. Carol would go with him.

"My dad was really tough on his students," Carol said, "and I think he got a charge out of embarrassing them. One of the first things you learn to get your pilot's license is to pre-check the plane."

Carol and her father would get to the airport an hour before any student. Carol would run around and say "Hi" to everyone while her father did the pre-check. When the students showed up, they also would do a pre-check.

"As they finished," Carol said, "my dad would look at me and say, 'Okay, Sam"—Carol's nickname was Sam—"you do to the pre-check.' I always found something wrong."

Maybe the plane was low on oil or a tire was low on air.

"My dad would look at his student," Carol said, "and he'd say something like, 'My eight-year-old can find things wrong, and you can't? You need to start over and find what she found.'"

"To me, it was like a game of hide and seek. But to them it was being shown up by a kid. When we finally got into the air, for the first half hour or so, I would stay quiet in the backseat of plane. After my dad stopped yelling at his student for doing something wrong and the student would start to feel as if he could handle the plane, it was time for me to have fun. My dad would turn and look at me and say, 'Okay, Sam, what do you want me to have him do?'"

"Stall the engine," Carol would say.

"The student would look at me with such fear," Carol said, "his eyes open big, his forehead all wrinkly. He'd shake his head back and forth fast. I would laugh at him."

She knew she was a devil. "I know my dad's students hated me," Carol said, "but for me it was the best roller coaster ride. I was a female Dennis the Menace."

# 8

---

One day, Kenneth took the family out on a boat.

"I know my dad saw something that got to him really really bad," Carol said. "He was yelling and cussing."

He slammed their boat in high gear, heading for a Coast Guard cutter and another boat that was passing something to the cutter.

"My mom was yelling and hitting my dad, yelling, 'Stop, Kenneth. Stop. We have the kids with us.'"

Carol knew that if they reached the two boats, they all would be in danger.

Kenneth took them home. The next weekend he went out with a couple of friends looking for any Coast Guard boat picking up drugs from an unidentified boat. On the first weekend in April, 1971, Sunday afternoon,

Jeanette, Carol's sister Linda, and Carol drove to the marina to pick up Kenneth and his friends. Carol felt the sea was "a little spooky" because it was so calm. Like glass.

There was no sign of Kenneth's boat. They waited for what seemed to Carol like hours.

"My dad was never late," Carol said. Jeanette became frantic, although she tried not to betray her fear.

Kenneth never returned.

All that was left of Kenneth's boat was the hatch to the engine room. The Mexican Coast Guard found the two guys Kenneth had been with floating in the water, murdered.

Jeanette kept trying to find out what had happened to Kenneth. She believed—against all evidence—that he was alive.

Over the years, Jeanette kept track of rumors of Coast Guard involvement with drug traffickers. In 1990, four Coast Guardsmen were convicted of helping drug smugglers and others were investigated.

"We have a few bad apples," Admiral Paul A. Yost, Jr., Commandant of the Coast Guard admitted. "I will ensure that they are prosecuted and punished."

Jeanette was cynical of official comments about Coast Guard-drug smuggler activities. A lot of cases were ignored or dismissed. When people claim some dishonest behavior was due to only a few "bad apples," it doesn't vindicate others: The old saying is "A few bad apples spoil the barrel." The *whole* barrel.

Early Sunday morning, Easter, Carol was awakened by a lady who stood at the foot of her bed.

"She had a long white dress with long brown hair," Carol said. "She told me I needed to get my sister and brother up and take them to church."

Carol went downstairs to get something to eat. Jeanette came into the kitchen and asked why Carol was up so early.

"I just said I was going to church and taking [siblings] Kendra and Kevin with me," Carol said. "My mom didn't think anything of it. It was Easter Sunday. Going to church was what one did.

"Back then I had an open heart to God," Carol said. "I even wanted to be a nun. My mom thought I was going to church with a lady from down the street."

Jeanette dressed Kendra and Kevin in their Sunday best. Carol took their hands and walked them to the church, which was on a hill possibly two miles away.

The sun was rising. Carol, Kendra, and Kevin got to the church parking lot, which was slightly higher than the building and gazed down at the church.

"I didn't understand it," Carol said. "It was Easter Sunday, and there were no cars."

Carol started to cry.

"Don't cry," said a woman behind her.

"But no one is here," Carol said.

"The doors will be open," the woman said.

Carol said, "Okay."

"Who are you talking to?" Kendra asked.

"I don't know," Carol said.

Only later would Carol understand the spirit who was coming to her was her grandmother. She thought it was an angel. And it was an angel—her grandmother had become an angel. Still holding Kendra and Kevin by the hand, Carol walked to the church doors.

"I let go of Kevin's hand and pulled on the door," Carol said.

It was locked.

Carol started to cry.

The woman said, "Don't cry."

"But," Carol said, "the door is locked."

The woman said, "The door will open for you."

Carol pulled on the door. It didn't move.

"Carol," the woman said, "look over there."

She was pointing to the left. A priest was walking toward them.

"Tell him about your dad," the woman said. Carol had been to this church a few times, but she didn't recognize this priest.

Children, the priest asked, What are you doing here so early?

"Our dad is missing," Carol said.

She told him what had happened to her dad

"We need God to find him for us," Carol said.

You want to pray? the priest asked.

"Yes," Carol said. "That's how God hears us."

All right, my children, the priest said, let's go inside, light some candles, and pray.

Carol said, "I didn't bring any money for the candles."

That's all right, my child, the priest said. I have this one.

And he produced a candle. After they lit candles and prayed, they went home, changed out of their best clothes, and went outside to play.

Carol went out to play and forgot all about her grandmother's spirit. But over the years, whenever Carol was at a low point, her grandmother's spirit appeared.

"She's one of the angels that always stays close to me," Carol explained.

"I don't recall telling the Father where we lived, but that afternoon he showed up at our house with a box of food," Carol said. "Now, this part I only know from what my mom's told me."

Mrs. Bishop, the priest said. I was visited by three angels this.

"You were?"

The oldest one, Sam, told me about your husband.

"Come in, Father. You said Sam told you about Kenneth?"

And I'm here to help in any way I can.

As they were talking, a man—a stranger —came to the door. He had papers that said Kenneth had been declared dead, and Jeanette and the children had only so much time to get out of military housing.

"When you're in the military, they take care of their own," Carol later said. "But, once a soldier is declared dead, the family has thirty days to get out of the military housing. It's like, 'Okay, here's your flag, now get out.'"

Even though Carol's father was missing and it is supposed to take seven years to legally declare a missing person dead, the military declared Kenneth dead within two weeks.

"And," Carol said, "that's the way it was."

Time to move out and on.

"My mom was handicapped," Carol said. "She had six kids and a grand-child on the way. Linda, my sister, was looking for my Dad. And the military was telling us to get out."

The priest helped them stay in the military housing months longer than they were supposed to, until the house they were going to move to was built.

Many years later, Carol asked her mom about the incident.

"She told me the priest was Father Charles," Carol said.

In June or July, 1973, while they were still living in Mira Mesa, Carol had lots of friends who lived in the cluster of about thirty homes.

"All the kids knew each other," Carol said, "and our house was the place to be. My mom always made the kids feel welcome. This one day, I ran into the house to get something to drink as four kids were running out."

The phone was ringing. Carol picked up the dining room phone and cupped her ear so she could hear whoever it was over the laughter and horseplay of the kids running in and out.

Breathless from laughing, Carol said, "Grand Central Station."

Hello? the man on the telephone said. Hello. What did you say?

"Grand Central Station," Carol said.

Is this the Bishop residence? the man asked.

"Yes," Carol said, "it is."

Did you answer the phone Grand Central Station? the man asked

"Yes," Carol said. "I did."

Did you know it's against the law to answer the phone that way? the man asked.

"No," Carol said. "I always answer the phone that way. It's always busy here."

The man on the phone said, This is President Nixon.

Another joker.

Is Mrs. Bishop there the man asked

"Sure," Carol said. "Hold on."

Carol shouted, "Mom. the phones for you. It's one of your friends."

After Jeanette got off the phone, she came out of her bedroom and said, "Carol Ann."

Trouble.

"Yes, ma'am," Carol said.

"How did you answer the phone?"

"The way I always do. Grand Central Station."

"Don't you ever answer the phone that way again," Jeanette said. "Do you know who that was?"

"He said he was President Nixon," Carol said. "But I didn't believe him."

"It was President Nixon," Jeanette said. "He was calling me about your dad." And about their staying on in military housing. Jeanette and Nixon spoke a number of times. "You just embarrassed me with the President of the United States."

"I'm sorry," Carol said.

"You're going to be sorry if you ever do that again," Jeanette said. "Now, go to your room."

"And that," Carol said, "is how I got in trouble with President Nixon."

# 9

"I'm a lot like my mom when it comes to certain things," Carol said. "I don't know what my mom was stirring up, but about two months after my Dad was gone I walked to the store with a friend."

As Carol and her friend were entering the grocery store, a man passed them going out.

"He was staring at me really strange," Carol said. "My friend and I stopped to see why." The man ran to his car, opened the door, sat behind the steering wheel, and looked down at something that, from a distance, looked like a picture.

"He looked at the picture, then looked at me," Carol said. "He did this about eight or nine times."

He got out of the car and walked to Carol.

"I was sent by your dad," he said.

He put his hand out and said, "Come with me."

Carol heard the woman's voice—her angels' voice— saying, "Run."

Carol and her friend ran—past the grocery store and into a hardware store—then behind the counter, trying to hide between the manager's legs. He could tell they were terrified.

The man came in and asked the manager if he had seen Carol and her friend come in.

The manager said no.

The man left.

The manager called the police.

A few months later, the first or second week in June, Carol was biking to her friend's house on the newly paved road when she flipped the bike, cut her chin, and hurt her chest.

Jeanette made Carol comfortable on the couch downstairs, then left the house with Carol's sister Linda to continue their search for Kenneth. Everyone else was upstairs, helping Carol's sister Karen get ready to graduate from grammar school.

Carol heard a knock on the door. She slipped off the couch and answered the knock. It was someone who claimed to know Kenneth. Carol let him in and lay back on the couch.

"The next thing I knew," Carol said, "he was on top of me."

She couldn't scream because of the stitches in her chin.

"I'm not sure how long it lasted," Carol said.

When it was over, he fell asleep in a chair.

Jeanette got home. The man who had raped Carol was still asleep. Carol took her mother into the kitchen and told her what had happened. MPs arrived, woke the rapist, and arrested him.

Carol's life was becoming a series of baffling events.

# 10

By 1969, Carol's mother was raising six kids by herself. Carol's oldest sister, Linda, sixteen and unmarried, was pregnant with a daughter.

"There was no stopping my mom." Carol said. "She did everything with us. She got us into softball, she got us into ice skating, she got us into horseback riding."

Carol had been with her boyfriend—Robert Laughlin—since the age of twelve when he saw her charge a kid she was fighting with even though she had a cast on her leg and crutches. He studied her softball form. He loved softball even more than he loved Simon and Garfunkel and Peter Frampton.

"Who is this crazy girl?" Robert asked around.

Robert and his parents had moved from Okinawa to Mira Mesa in 1974. Before school started in the fall, Robert asked Carol to go steady. Carol happily accepted.

Jeanette and the rest of the family welcomed Robert. At night, afraid Carol and her family may have been targeted by whoever killed Kenneth's companions (and maybe Kenneth), Robert would walk Carol home from wherever she was. Sometimes, he'd walk Kendra home, too. He spent more and more time at Carol's house.

Robert's dad was dead set against his son's relationship with Carol. He knew about Kenneth—and Carol's uncle Ronald, who was rumored to be in the CIA—and told Robert not to have anything to do with Carol or her family. Robert ignored his father's warning.

"My dad knew something he wasn't telling me," Robert said.

His father (who was a Marine) had checked with friends at CIC (The United States Army Criminal Investigation Command, which investigates crimes committed by the United States military), tracking Kenneth and confirming that a Mexican ship was loading drugs onto a Coast Guard cutter that would take the drugs to the shore.

When Kenneth disappeared, Robert heard many conflicting stories.

"I'd heard someone told Carol's dad to forget what he had seen," Robert said. "But that wasn't likely to scare Carol's dad off."

Carol caught her uncle Ronald—her mother's brother, who maybe was in the CIA—doing drugs in her house. He drove a Cadillac. Once when Ronald popped his trunk, she saw guns. To avoid certain members of their family—like her brother Ronald?—Jeanette always had an unlisted number. They all did, including Carol and her siblings. But people always found out where they lived.

Seven years or so after Kenneth disappeared, Carol, Kendra, and Robert were at the pool at Kendra's apartment, swimming, sunbathing, fooling around. When they had left the apartment, they had locked up. When they went back, they found the door broken in. There was some money on the bar, which was untouched. Nothing was taken except every family picture. It wasn't a typical robbery.

That unnerved Kendra so much that she left California and moved to Maryland. She was working one day at BWI, Baltimore International Airport, at one of the stands. All day long, there was a page for a Kenneth Elmer Bishop, not a common name. Kendra couldn't leave her post. When she got off, she couldn't find out anything about the page. She hurried home and told her sister, Linda.

"Linda called up the airport and asked for the paging department. She wanted to know if a Kenneth Elmer Bishop had been paged," Carol said. "The response was, "Oh my gosh, yes, all day long.""

Years after, in April, 1981, there was the letter—or rather an envelope, which was sent to Carol's mother Jeanette. There was no return address. Inside was a clipping from a North African newspaper. There was a photograph of half a dozen men in the French Foreign Legion. One face was circled. It looked to Janette like it was her husband, Kenneth Elmer Bishop.

Maybe trying to protect his family from whomever he had been chasing in the waters off California, Kenneth had disappeared into the Foreign Legion among Legionnaires from 140 countries.

# 11

For what was supposed to be Robert's junior year in high school, Robert's dad was transferred to Okinawa. Robert didn't want to go to Japan. His dad told him if he left the house to go his own way not to come back.

Robert's stepmother took him to Hammondsport, which one website calls "America's Coolest Small Town." It has a population of eight hundred people and was on Keuka Lake, one of the five Finger Lakes in upstate New York. Wine country. Robert couldn't wait to see snow. He arrived in time for a storm that was considered the worst in a decade.

"I saw snow, all right," Robert said. "It was so cold cars were driving out on the frozen lake."

After a year, Robert returned to Mira Mesa and moved in with Carol's family.

In 1980, Carol and Robert set a date to get married in San Diego's Balboa Park. They put down a deposit for a wedding dinner.

But, during a softball game, Carol (who was catcher) walked up to Robert (who was behind the backstop), said, "I'm pregnant," and walked back to her position.

Instead of a big wedding, they were married on July 19, 1981, by a Baptist minister at Jeanette's home.

After the wedding ceremony, Robert in his tuxedo and Carol, bunching her wedding dress under her so she could sit on it, climbed on Carol's peddle-start Peugeot moped and sailed off.

Carol had a son, Kenneth. Kenny.

"We had a kid before we had a relationship," Carol said.

In her wedding vows, Carol promised "to love, honor, and obey."

"I'm pretty sure she promised 'to obey,'" Robert said, "but I don't think anyone can imagine Carol obeying anyone. Anyway, no one snickered."

A few months later, they moved to Texas, where Robert had family in Greenville. Carol's sister, Karen, was living there as well.

"Kenny was still in diapers," Carol said.

Not long after Kenny was born, Carol had a daughter, Kimberly.

Kimberly was a premie. When she was born in June of 1982, she weighed five pounds three ounces. In the first days, she lost half her body weight, so she was in the hospital for four months.

# 12

---

Carol didn't know about her mom's second marriage, because she was in Mexico. Carol was concerned—she didn't want Jeanette to lose her military benefits—but she liked Jeanette's new husband, Willem Lunshof.

In August 1983, Robert joined the Army for a three-year tour.

"We had rough patches," Carol said about her marriage, which didn't last.

Carol said she wanted a divorce.

"I was complaisant," Robert said.

He went along with her.

"We started dating at twelve," Robert said. "We outgrew each other."

"No animosity," Carol agreed. "No lawyers."

They continued to be friends. And, whenever things got tough, Carol would consult him.

In 1989, they separated.

"I'm not sure when we got divorced," Carol said. "I think it was in 1991 or 1992."

After the divorce, Carol moved to Connecticut, where one of her sisters was living in Shalton.

"Wherever she went, Carol went," Robert said.

Carol got a place in Danbury, Connecticut, where she got a job at Burger King. And then at Boston Market. She started as a cashier, bused the dining room, became shift supervisor, then manager, then general manager.

"I just kept learning and learning," Carol said.

Robert reappeared. Carol unsuccessfully tried to make the marriage work again. Robert ended up moving to North Carolina.

"Back then, when I was working," Carol said, "I was really cocky, because my mom taught me, 'Don't expect other people to do the job. You do it yourself, until it's done right. And, if other people have to do it, you just make sure it's done right.'"

"If you treat your employees with respect and dignity," Carol said, "they're going to treat you with respect and dignity."

She drove employees home in her red Mustang convertible. No matter what the weather, even in the middle of winter, she always had the top down.

Management—which came around all the time, checking—gave her a triple-A rating, which was hard to get. Once, when Carol went on a vacation, the CEO Jeff Kindell—who was touring—called her and asked, "Why do you have a homeless man cleaning out your dumpster?"

"Well," Carol said, "he was bothering my customers for food to eat, so I went out and talked to him. I said, 'You can't do that.'"

She made a deal with him. If he cleaned the dumpster, Carol would feed him twice a day.

He said he was good with that.

Carol gave him a shirt and fed him as she had promised. And he kept the dumpster clean. Win-win.

At a Boston Market conference in Las Vegas, Kindell gave a speech to the assembled Boston Market employees. He told them that if they wanted a good store, call Carol; then he gave out her cell phone number. Carol started getting calls from all over—Texas, Massachusetts, New York—asking her to visit a store and fix whatever was wrong. The first thing she would do is to tell the employees, "You guys aren't doing anything wrong. The management is. You just haven't been trained right. You want to do a good job, and I'm going to make sure you're able to. I'm going to give you the right stuff to do it, and I'm going to show you how. But first, I've got to teach these guys in management how to do their jobs, and how to teach, and how to treat you."

Carol married again. She refuses to mention her ex's name—just like Robert, who won't mention it either.

"I only married him because it was his mother's dying wish to see him married," Carol said.

The marriage was a disaster.

"That guy was an asshole," Robert said.

Carol arranged to get transferred to Baltimore's Boston Market office.

Because her second husband—now ex-husband—kept driving down to see her, Carol told Boston Markets not to list her name on her office door. She also went back to her maiden name.

And then she met Gary.

# 13

On their first long trip together, Gary and Carol went to Ocean City, Maryland. They strolled the Boardwalk and walked along the beach collecting sea shells, which they later put on Stevie's and Peggy's (Gary's mom) graves. They watched the seagulls dive toward the water. At bars, Gary drank Grey Goose vodka, and Carol drank rum and Cokes. They shopped for clothes, ate Thrasher's French fries and crabs. Dozens of crabs. Gary loved crabs.

But mostly they spent a lot of time in their room. They loved room service and usually had breakfast and dinner inside. They'd sit on their terrace watching the dolphins swim in one direction in the morning and swim in the other direction in the evening. Like commuters. When there was a lunar eclipse, they spent the night on the terrace, taking over two hundred pictures with Gary's camera.

On the beach, in the clubs, and in their room, Gary kept his two phones close.

"Two of everything," Carol said.

Posting bonds was a 24/7 job even if David covered for Gary in his absence.

After eight days, when Gary went to check out, he found that Carol had already paid the bill.

"We will always be 50/50," Carol said.

# 14

Soon after they got home, on March 12, 2005, they headed out again to a wedding in Columbus, Maryland. Carol's niece—Candace—was getting married.

On the way there, Gary pulled over to the side of the road and asked Carol, "How about making it a double wedding?"

They got the giggles. But, through the laughter, Gary said he was being serious. He wanted to marry her, but he didn't want her answer until after the celebration, so during the reception he would have a chance to ask Carol's step-father, Willem, for her hand. He blessed their union.

Gary and Carol planned to have a big wedding. They were going to have the reception at the Cantina. Carol bought her dress and Gary got his tuxedo.

On April 26, Gary told Carol he didn't want to wait anymore. They could have a big reception later at the Cantina. Carol was excited by the drama of it. It was almost like eloping. On May 1, Carol put on a long dress (not the wedding dress she had bought). Gary put on a business suit, not his tux. They went to City Hall, where they had a simple wedding. Gary kept his eyes averted until he repeated until death do us part. Then, Gary looked the justice full in the face.

After leaving City Hall, Gary and Carol followed a rainbow that seemed to end at a Taco Bell, where they stopped for a meal.

At first, they didn't tell anyone at the Cantina. Gary wanted their marriage to be just between the two of them until the big wedding reception. But the big wedding reception never came. Gary's father—Sonny—passed away.

On October 10, 2011, Carol's best friend Sindie died at Johns Hopkins Hospital in Baltimore. Carol had no warning. She never had a chance to tell Sindie her secret.

# 15

One night, in Princess George County, a rough area near Washington, D.C., when Carol was taking the local Boston Market's receipts to the bank, she was attacked. There were about fifteen people, including men, watching the attack. Not one helped as the thug beat Carol up.

Carol fought back.

"I got him a couple good times," she said.

He started running. Carol ran after him, shouting to the onlookers, "Get the son of a bitch. I'm not done."

It was obvious Carol was seriously hurt. Someone called the cops and an ambulance.

Someone else asked, How much did he get?

"What are you talking about?" Carol asked.

He robbed you, right? the guy said.

Carol opened up her pants and started pulling out deposit after deposit, $12,000 to $15,000.

"Ain't nobody going down my pants," Carol said.

Carrying loose bills was against company policy. You're supposed to put it in a bag. In a bag? Really? Carol figured, that was saying, "Hey, rob me." She always carried an empty dummy bag. The mugger didn't get a penny.

Carol had started carrying a dummy since 2003, when she'd worked in Bridgeport, Connecticut, in an area close to the DMV, which people called Father Panic.

Even ambulance drivers avoided the neighborhood.

Carol was proud of going there, proud of being a woman who went there.

Gary called her and asked, "How's work going?"

Carol said, "I'm not at work. I'm at the hospital."

They x-rayed her. She had nerve damage from her C-3 through her C-7 vertebrae and damage on the left side of her neck. Her left arm was in bad shape.

As soon as she was finished with the exam, she went home, because she had trainees who were getting ready to take their final exam. While Carol was recuperating, she met with the trainees in her apartment. Since she didn't have to do any physical work, Carol cut her medical leave short and went back to the store.

Gary kept close tabs on her. If she was working a double shift and was closing, taking the day's receipts to the bank, Gary showed up, no matter what store it was, no matter what city. Carrying his Glock. When the doctors diagnosed Carol as having permanent nerve damage from the beating, Gary devoted himself to taking care of her.

# 16

Around 2000, when Gary was thirty-three years old he went in for a colonoscopy, a regular checkup, and the doctor—the same one who had looked at Gary years earlier when he'd been diagnosed as having Crohn's Disease—noticed some new inflammation. For six months, Gary took Remicade. His inflammation—and the pain—went away, except for one little tiny spot that the doctor didn't like the look of. He left it up to Gary whether to continue the medication or to have surgery to cut it out.

"Go ahead," Gary said. "Take it out."

After that surgery, Gary felt healthier than he ever had before. He had no more pain in his gut—until 2011, when Carol found Gary sitting on the couch, rocking.

All week, she watched Gary suffering. He was constantly in the bathroom. He was dry heaving. He wouldn't come to bed. He wasn't eating. When he was alone, he moaned. He lost his temper over small things. Carol thought he was starting to snap. She called David and said, "Your brother is sick, and he won't do anything, or go to the hospital. Can you come over?"

When the ambulance Carol called got to their house, the EMS workers told Carol that Gary was having a heart attack. They were taking him to Sinai, the hospital where Gary had been born. When Carol got to the hospital, they wouldn't let her into the Emergency Room, where they had taken him, until they had checked a couple of things out. A friendly nurse told Carol that if she had ridden in the ambulance with him, she could have stayed with her husband—not information Carol expected to need again.

When she finally got to Gary—who by now was no longer in his favorite holey T-shirt but in a hospital gown—he told her the doctors had ruled out a heart attack and had diagnosed him as suffering from a Crohn's Disease flare up.

"They're looking at the wrong thing," Gary told Carol.

His pain was in his left upper quadrant. Gary kept saying that his Crohn's presented in the lower part of his belly, right below his belly button and not where his present pain was. Crohn's pain is typically crampy, which Gary did not have. Maybe it was colitis, but the doctors never suggested colitis.

Crohn's can affect any part of the digestion system from the throat to the anus. Stress can exacerbate Crohn's. Eating the poppy seeds from a bagel can also exacerbate Crohn's. Gary had a history of Crohn's, the doctors figured, so this must be Crohn's.

The first test they did (for the bacteria C. *difficile*, an infection of the bowel, especially in people who have been treated with antibiotics) came back negative. Five other people on the floor had C. diff, so they did a second test, which came back positive.

"Which also led the doctors to assume it was Crohn's," Carol said.

Gary also had an elevated white count, which is consistent with an infection, possibly Crohn's.

In Carol's opinion, from the start, the doctors focused on Crohn's to the exclusion of other possibilities: "They didn't do due diligence," Carol said. "They didn't do an endoscopy on him to see what was going on in the upper part of his intestinal and stomach area. If they did, I wouldn't be talking to you right now. I would be talking to my husband."

Gary started yelling, "This isn't my Crohn's."

He begged Carol to set them straight. But the doctors went a different way. They gave him steroids, which is one of the treatments for Crohn's Disease, including Prednisone and Toradol, which, according to some experts could have made Gary's condition worse.

"Gary didn't have Crohn's," Carol said. "He had an ulcer. Which perforated."

And doomed Gary to death.

# Part Two

---

# Not On My Watch

## 17

Gary's gut hurt when he took a breath. The pain was ten out of ten. But he couldn't take pain medication when his blood pressure was low.

"And," Carol said, "there were times he was so afraid of being in pain, that it didn't matter how much pain medicine you gave him."

Gary's ulcer was in his duodenum, where the stomach attaches to the small intestine. The pain radiated to his chest. He came to Sinai Hospital Emergency Room on May 12 about 11:16 at night and was seen by an emergency room physician, who recorded Gary's complaints as severe pain in the left upper quadrant that got worse when he breathed or changed position. The doctor confirmed that when he pressed Gary's belly the area was "tender."

He ordered blood work and a CAT scan of Gary's abdomen and pelvis. Carol worried that doctors were not paying sufficient attention to Gary's complaint that the pain radiated to his chest.

After examining Gary's CAT scan, another doctor—Dr. Suzette Johnson-Futrell—suspected the inflammation in Gary's colon was related to Crohn's Disease, partly because of Gary's history.

On May 13, Dr. Johnson-Futrell admitted Gary to the hospital. She requested a consult with a gastrointestinal specialist from Woodholme Gastroenterology, an established firm in Pikesville that had been founded in 1986. She wanted someone with GI expertise to examine Gary. That was Dr. Todd Heller.

In 1980, Heller graduated <u>Summa Cum Laude</u> from Yeshiva College in New York City. In 1984, got his medical degree from Albert Einstein College at Yeshiva. From 1984 to 1987, he did his residency in the Bronx at Montefiore Hospital. In 1989, he got a fellowship at St. Luke's Hospital in New York City to further study gastroenterology—an admirable record.

Heller saw Gary on the 14th, around 9 a.m.

Heller had short hair, wore dark framed glasses, and had a ready smile. He had a commanding and comforting presence.

Carol trusted him, at first.

Years before, in 2000, Heller had treated Gary for his Crohn's, but he didn't recall Gary in 2011. He reviewed Gary's medical records and asked Gary what was going on, and about Gary's past medical history. He did a physical examination and went over the previous diagnostic studies, and wrote a report back to Dr. Johnson-Futrell, who had requested this consult, telling her about his findings and his recommendations.

Even though Gary kept telling Heller that the pain did not feel like his previous Crohn's, which had been in the lower right quadrant and not where the pain was now, in the upper left quadrant, and even though Heller confirmed that Gary's "tenderness" was in the upper left quadrant, Heller was inclined to agree with Johnson-Futrell's diagnosis: Crohn's.

The final report of the CAT scan, unlike that preliminary interpretation, indicated no inflammation. The radiologist who issued that final report stated, "Findings do not suggest active disease."

Despite that, when Heller wrote his note to Johnson-Futrell, he indicated that what was going on here was Crohn's Disease, and as a result, he recommended to Johnson-Futrell that they continue to give Gary steroids, which is one of the treatments for Crohn's Disease—and which many doctors say can make ulcers worse.

# 18

Heller wanted Gary to have a colonoscopy, a large bowel study, mostly of the lower abdomen. Heller did not order any testing to evaluate the upper left quadrant, or the upper half, where Gary indicated he had pain. He did not do any tests to evaluate Gary's esophagus, stomach, gallbladder, pancreas, and duodenum; no endoscopy, which, according to other doctors, might have revealed Gary's ulcer.

On the next day, May 15, Dr. Heller got the results of the tests he had ordered. There was no sign of active Crohn's.

"I put doctors on pedestals back then," Carol said. "I assumed they knew what they were doing."

Heller concluded that Gary was suffering from a Crohn's flare-up.

On May 17, Gary was discharged—partly because, Carol was convinced, "Gary didn't have the proper medical insurance."

Get out, like the government had told Jeanette about military housing after Carol's father had disappeared.

Gary's ulcer had been undiagnosed and untreated.

# 19

Eight days later, on May 25, 2011, Carol called another ambulance. Gary's pain was still eight out of ten, ten out of ten. He felt as if there was a gas bubble in his abdomen.

He couldn't go back to Sinai, Carol was told, because they had no beds available in the ER. She suspected the real reason had to do with Gary's insufficient insurance.

The ambulance took Gary to Northwest Hospital on Liberty Road in Randallstown.

Again, Carol followed Gary's ambulance. Again, she ran red lights. Again, the EMS Techs figured Gary was suffering from a heart attack.

Northwest was "where things got really bad," Carol said. "That's where he got opened up for the first time."

In the emergency room, Gary complained about his left side abdominal pain. The doctors said he was guarding: when someone pressed on Gary's abdomen, he tensed his muscles in reaction to the pain.

Gary was admitted to the hospital and put on "nothing by mouth," or NPO. A doctor in the radiology department consulted with Dr. Steven Epstein.

Like Dr. Heller, Dr. Epstein got his undergraduate degree Summa Cum Laude at Union College in Schenectady, New York, in 1998. He had been an excellent student. In 2002, he went to medical school at the University of Maryland, where he did his internship and residency. About 10 to 20 percent of Epstein's patients suffered from Crohn's Disease. He also was experienced in treating peptic ulcers, which he explained were more common than Crohn's.

On May 26, Dr. Epstein examined Gary, who seemed to be a typical case, one of many unmemorable patients.

In general, Dr. Epstein's note said, the patient is walking around the room, appearing comfortable, in no acute distress.

Dr. Epstein didn't order an upper endoscopy or any testing of Gary's upper gastrointestinal tract, which might have revealed Gary's ulcer.

Dr. Epstein seemed to agree with the charts from Sinai that Gary was suffering from Crohn's, although the charts also reported that Gary was complaining about pain in his left upper quadrant—which many medical experts agree is not consistent with a diagnosis of Crohn's.

At the time, Carol was fighting the government about getting Gary a disability claim. The doctors speculated that Carol's fight may have exacerbated Gary's stress, which can trigger Crohn's flares.

On May 28, just after midnight, 12:38, about thirty-three hours after Dr. Epstein had seen Gary, Gary's pain became unbearable. Possibly during the early morning hours of May 28, Gary's ulcer perforated his bowel wall and allowed gastric content to seep into his abdomen.

A physician's assistant noted Gary's pain was in the upper right quadrant. His blood pressure dropped. He was diaphoretic—pouring sweat. He had none of the normal sounds a bowel makes when it's working properly. The medical records described Gary as being in distress. He developed lactic acidosis; his tissues and organs were not getting enough oxygen.

Gary had exploratory surgery by a different doctor, a surgeon, who noticed that in the lower right quadrant, Gary's intestines didn't look normal, partly because of Gary's previous Crohn's operation in 2000.

The surgeon cut out a piece of Gary's bowel, which he sent to a hospital pathologist, who didn't find any inflammation.

# 20

Gary's brother, David, and his wife, Stacey, were on vacation, on a beach in Ocean City when David got a call from Carol, telling him to come home immediately. Gary was in the hospital with severe pain in his gut.

They had come in two cars. David took off immediately in one. Stacey packed and checked out of the hotel where they were staying and followed in the other.

When Stacey got to the hospital, she was shocked by Gary's condition. He was drawn and obviously in pain. But Gary joked about his condition, partly to put others at ease. That was typical of Gary.

"Being a nurse," Stacey said, "I've seen a lot."

But Gary struck her as being in serious trouble. She measured the surgical incision in Gary's belly: one and a half by nine inches.

Gary was sitting in his hospital room chair when he started to bleed out. Blood was seeping from every orifice.

Carol and David tried to distract Gary from what was happening as they mopped it up.

Gary was rushed back into surgery, where the doctors repaired the leaks. They closed him up as best they could.

"The doctor is telling us, 'we have to put a colostomy bag on your brother,'" David said, "and we said go ahead."

When Gary came out of surgery, he grabbed David and said, "They messed up. They messed up."

# 21

Gary was septic, which decreased his blood supply, which prevented the anastomosis (a surgical connection) that the surgeon had created in the first operation from healing. It reopened, letting more gastro content into Gary's abdomen. The doctors decided not to close Gary back up so he could heal. Instead, they put him in the Intensive Care Unit.

At some point, Gary noticed he was wearing the wrong hospital identification bracelet. He told Carol, who tried to find out what the other Gary Stern was in for to make sure her Gary wasn't being treated for what the other Gary suffered from.

And vice versa.

Carol tried to get answers, but it was hard. Her trust in doctors was quickly eroding. She began to believe they were fallible, even defensive.

The other Gary was suffering from a heart condition.

"To this day," Carol said, "I still get calls to pay for the other Stern."

Up until then, Gary trusted the doctors.

"It's like a car mechanic saying you need brakes," Gary said. "So you get brakes."

On June 13, nineteen days after Gary entered Northwest, the surgeon arranged to transfer him back to Sinai Hospital, where he thought Gary could get better help.

Gary had become complicated, as the doctors phrased it.

# 22

The night before Gary was to be moved back to Sinai, Carol was giving Gary a sponge bath. She noticed one of Gary's JP [Jackson-Pratt] tubes—which drained internal fluids from his body—had green matter in it. She had no idea what it meant. The next morning, she waited to tell the doctors what she had seen, but they didn't show up. She couldn't ask.

"It was a beautiful sunny day," Carol said, "but Gary couldn't enjoy it. He was in too much pain and terrified of what was going on with his body."

At 5:30 p.m., he was finally moved.

Carol followed the ambulance in the van, running another red light. Of course.

At Sinai, Gary was put in the IMC [Intermediate Care] floor, room 27. All the rooms were huge and clean. Gary's was close to the nurses' station.

At 6:30 at night, there was a shift change. No one appeared.

Carol could see that Gary was getting uncomfortable. Close to 7, and still no one had come in. Gary started moaning.

"What's going on," Carol asked.

"I need to go to the bathroom," Gary said.

Carol pushed the call button.

No one came.

Carol looked into the hall. She didn't see anyone.

Gary was increasingly uncomfortable.

Carol decided to take him herself. She managed to get Gary sitting on the side of the bed, legs hanging over, hoping someone would come in.

The bed was fifteen feet from the bathroom.

Gary hadn't stood up since his last surgery. It took a little bit. Finally, Carol had Gary standing. He was shaky, so Carol put both of Gary's arms on her shoulders. He was too weak to lift his head, which drooped onto Carol's chest. Carol started silently praying, "Please, Lord, help me get Gary to the bathroom."

Carol heard a voice, but it wasn't her inner voice this time. It was Gary, but so weak Carol could hardly hear him.

"Carol! Carol!" Gary said. "I think I'm dying! I can feel it. I am dying."

Carol couldn't breathe.

"No, no, this is not happening," she said.

Another voice.

This time it wasn't Gary. It was her inner voice, which said, *"Don't let him give up."*

Carol leaned over so she could see Gary's eyes and he could see hers.

"You're not going to die!" Carol said. "Not on my watch."

Gary sat on the toilet. Carol could hear liquid pouring out of Gary.

Carol thought it went on for at least five minutes.

"Wow, Gary," Carol said. "You really had to go."

"I guess so," Gary said. "I think I'm done."

Carol bent down to make sure. What she saw was horrifying. Gary wasn't going to the bathroom. Green liquid was pouring out of his JP tube, from the incision above his penis.

Carol looked at Gary's beautiful brown eyes.

"I can't lose him," she thought. "Gary is the perfect man for me."

Carol didn't want Gary to know what was going on.

"I told him he might not be done yet," Carol said, to keep him from getting up and seeing what had happened.

She pushed the bathroom call button.

"Nurses seem to come in faster," Carol said, "when you push the button in the bathroom."

Within a few moments, an assistant nurse came. Carol told her to stay with Gary, but not to let him see what was in the toilet bowl. She hurried to the nurses' station and pounded her hand on the counter, yelling, "Get me my husband's doctor. Get me my husband's nurse. Get me the charge nurse. Now!"

She was terrified. She didn't understand why no doctors had been to see Gary yet. She didn't know what the hell was going on.

By the time everyone—doctors and nurses— had arrived, Carol was no longer terrified. She was pissed.

"You two get in my husband's room," Carol told two nurses. "Get him cleaned up. Get him back into bed. And he is *not* to see his body. You are *not* to comment on what you see until you're out of his room."

Carol told a third nurse, "You go get my husband some pain medication. Some Ativan."

"You need to put the orders in," Carol told the doctor. "You need to examine my husband. Then, we can go into the hall, you can tell me what the hell is going on."

After the examination, the doctor—who turned out to be a PA (a physician's assistant)—told Carol that Gary was septic and would be going to the OR at seven the next morning.

Carol couldn't sleep that night. She just sat in a chair watching Gary.

She remembered the story Gary used to tell her about when he drove at a NASCAR race and was black flagged for going too fast. She thought about how he was always running fast to do something. Anything. Everything. And, now, he was just lying in that bed, expecting to die. It was that night Carol made up her mind to learn everything she could about what was going on with Gary's body.

She learned everything about Gary's medications, how to read and understand blood labs, learning what vitals were supposed to be and what it meant if they were not in the normal range.

Carol learned medical terminology, "so I could speak at their levels," she said. "That's why doctors and nurses would ask me where I had practiced medicine. I would ask them had they done this, had they tried that? Because I had looked it up."

# 23

At Sinai, on June 14, Gary was back in surgery. Among other procedures, the surgeon cleaned up the mess inside Gary, including a fistula [an opening between two internal organs or between an internal organ and the outside of the body]. He cut out more of Gary's bowel, creating an ostomy: a drain from the inside to the outside of a body]. Gary's bowel was diverted through his skin and into a bag.

Carol ran into the head of the hospital in the elevator. She suppressed the urge to bawl him out.

Carol's military mother taught Carol to always go up the chain of command—which she did, until she got a <u>no</u>. Then, she went higher.

But confronting the head of the hospital—what was the point?

Hospitals are bureaucracies, in which patients can only be profit-making cogs. At the same time they are places for healing, in which helping patients get better is the only thing that matters.

Gary was just one of hundreds.

But Gary was Carol's husband. One of one. Unique. As all patients are.

The head of the hospital gave Carol his card.

"If you ever have any trouble," he said, "you give me a call."

Despite Gary's pain, he managed to get his sense of humor back. Sinai is a teaching hospital, so every day at 5 a.m. the doctors would do rounds, each with an entourage of third-year medical students and interns. When anyone came to visit, Gary would pretend to be the doctor and say, "You have temperature. No temperature. Write this down. Temperature okay."

The doctors would take Carol into the hall, scratching their heads and saying they didn't understand why Gary's not running a temperature, that his white count was very high. They told her Gary was going to die.

"Gary never played by the rules," Carol said.

One day Gary's nurse (who usually worked in the ICU cardiology unit) noticed that Gary's heart rate was way too high. When the surgeon came in, she talked him into moving Gary to the ICU.

That afternoon, David and Stacey visited Gary in the ICU room—which only allowed two people in at a time—and the surgeon stopped by. David called Carol and said she had to come. Immediately. When Carol arrived, she overheard the surgeon telling David that he was going to take Gary back to surgery.

"If you do," David said, "I will cut *you* open."

Carol laughed.

The surgeon looked at her.

"You heard the man," Carol said. "No more surgeries."

The next day, the surgeon told Carol he needed to have another doctor come in for a consultation. To back him up, Carol figured. He told her Gary needed surgery because his white blood cell count was 77,000. People only have a white cell count that high when they're suffering from cancer.

The consulting doctor examined Gary and said that Gary did not have cancer. But he was septic. They treated him and Gary responded. In a few days, Gary was sent back to the Intermediate Care Unit.

Carol started taking the pictures of Gary's abdomen, so she could show the doctors.

"When a doctor came in the next day after I showed him the pictures, the hospital gave Gary a plate of French fries and fried chicken."

Carol picked up the plate.

"What are you doing?" Gary asked.

Carol threw the plate at the door.

To the nurse, she said, "He has an intestinal fistula. Why am I having to tell you this? Why are you feeding my husband?"

Gary hadn't eaten anything in six weeks.

"Why," Carol asked, "didn't they start him on a soft diet of broth and Jell-O, a clear liquid diet?"

Fried chicken and French fries?

"I'm not a medical expert," Carol said, "but I knew better than to feed my husband fried chicken and French fries."

They put in a central line, which goes into a big vein close to the heart. "Because it's closer to the heart," Carol said, "medication has to be dripped at a slower rate. You can't have way too much going to your heart at one time."

Carol would sleep in a chair in Gary's room, terrified of what could or would happen to Gary if she wasn't right there. She would watch Gary suffer in pain, getting depressed.

She would sit there thinking, *what could I do?*

First things first: pray.

Carol would listen to Gary moan.

It would go on for hours, sometimes days.

She would sit there and pray for the pain to stop, for Gary to smile again,

Carol remembered Gary; the way he would smile when they decorated the house for Christmas; the smile on his face when he took her hand and walked her onto the dance floor.

Carol would think about the time he slid over the hood of a moving car to get to her because he saw five men hassling her.

She needed to do something, but what? She couldn't do anything about the pain but maybe she could do something about the depression, but what? Gary couldn't eat, he couldn't get up.

The answer: Jade, Carol's granddaughter, Kenny's daughter, coming for a visit. But Jade was in school.

So, what?

Carol thought about it, then prayed some more. Carol got a phone call from her daughter, Kimberly, who wanted to come to Baltimore with her daughter Nadilla —to see Gary.

*Wow,* Carol thought, *Gary loves babies and he hadn't met Nadilla yet.* Another of Carol's granddaughters. *This should work,* she thought.

Which it did for a few days.

# 24

The nurses were telling Carol to get Gary into a bigger hospital.

A *red flag,* Carol thought.

The surgeon agreed. He told Carol that Gary needed to be transferred, possibly to Johns Hopkins.

"Gary needs to go to the University of Maryland," Carol said.

She had done her homework.

The University of Maryland Hospital didn't have a bed available.

Do you have any idea when? Carol asked.

No, the surgeon said. Is there anything else I can do for you two?

Yes, Carol said. The dogs. Carol wanted to take Gary outside so he could see his dogs, especially Butchy.

I don't know if we can do that, the surgeon said.

*I'm going to make it happen*, Carol said to herself. "Who would know?" Carol said to the surgeon.

Carol told the charge nurse.

"I need to take Gary outside to see his dogs."

He can't leave the floor, the charge nurse said. Gary's on a heart monitor.

"So," Carol said, "just take it off."

We can't do that, the charge nurse said. All patients on IMC have to be monitored at all times.

"I'll monitor him," Carol said.

It's against policy, the charge nurse said. It's not possible.

"Okay," Carol told the nurse. "I'll take care of it."

Good luck, the nurse said. Later that day Carol ran into Kelly, another charge nurse, one who had taken care of Gary.

"I need your help with something I was told I can't do," Carol said. "You know that Gary is being transferred to UMD. Gary is really nervous about the move, very depressed."

Would you like me to talk to him? Kelly asked.

"I need you to help me get him outside," Carol said, "so he can see his dogs."

That's against policy, Kelly said.

"I heard," Carol said.

But, Kelly said, it is possible. Kelly explained they needed to get a doctor to sign off on the idea. Someone would have to leave the floor with him.

That's going to be really hard, Kelly said, because we always have more than one patient.

"Getting the doctor to sign off will be easy," Carol said.

Carol went to the back of the hospital next to the cafeteria's outside tables to smoke and call David, who said he would pick up the dogs. As Carol ended the call, one of the physician's assistants approached her. Carol suspected she was about to be manipulated.

How is Mr. Stern doing today? the physician's assistant asked.

"He's depressed and nervous about the move," Carol said.

Is there anything I can do?

"As a matter of fact, there may be. Are you working tomorrow?"

Yes, I am.

"Gary has really been missing his dogs, so I want to surprise him and bring the dogs up here, so Gary can spend some time with them. But the policy won't let him come outside without someone with him."

I'm having lunch out here tomorrow at about one o'clock, so I can be here.

Carol was surprised. The physician's assistant had come not to manipulate but to help.

Carol blessed her, went back upstairs, and found Kelly—"who kept her word to help," Carol said.

The next day Carol removed Gary's heart monitor and took him downstairs and outside.

Gary had no idea what was going on. Carol wheeled him outside. Stacey handed him some dog treats. Gary looked confused—and then he saw David and the dogs.

For an hour, Gary—in his wheelchair with a plastic bag protecting his stomach—Carol, David, and Stacey took the dogs for a walk.

# 25

At the beginning of August, Gary was still waiting to be transferred to the University of Maryland Hospital. He was terrified of the move. Carol assured him it was the right thing to do. She needed to get Gary's spirits up. Maybe the move could eventually do it.

Carol wasn't eating, wasn't sleeping.

David was doing everything he could, but Carol needed more help.

She called Kenny, her son from her first marriage.

"Anytime Gary and I needed Kenny," Carol said, "he would drop whatever he was doing and come" and would stay long enough to enable Carol to work on Medicare and Medicaid and other ways of trying to get medical coverage.

The wound nurse came in to change Gary's dressing.

How can you stay with Gary? a nurse asked Carol. He yells at you so much.

"He's not yelling at me," Carol explained, "he's yelling at the situation."

Another nurse, Kim, asked Carol if she was homeless because she never left Gary's room.

"They allowed Carol to sleep in the room," David said. "Gary could get nasty if she wasn't there. He screamed at the doctors."

He threw things at the doctors. Told them to get the hell out.

A lot of doctors and nurses wouldn't come to Gary's room.

"But good people stayed involved," Carol said. "Not everyone was an idiot. Some were worried about a lawsuit."

"It was the big talk on the IMC [intermediate care] floor," Carol said. "By this time, all the doctors started telling me they didn't know what to do. Gary was dying, and they were shrugging their shoulders."

# 26

In August 2011, Gary was transferred to the University of Maryland Hospital.

The University of Maryland Hospital is big. The main building was built out of brick in the mid-1800s. When they needed to expand, they built around the hospital and then connected the buildings together. Carol thought it seemed like a maze—both physically and bureaucratically – through which she had to find her way.

She was Theseus. Gary's death was the Minotaur she had to defeat.

In some areas of the hospital, even though you're inside, it looks as if you're outside. Carol would usually go through the revolving door at the side entrance. It reminded Carol of a mall with no stores.

"Past the offices and the trees," Carol said, "you can see a small cookie store. You can walk past it to the right about fifty yards to the front of the hospital; and, if you turn to the left and walk ten yards, you see a building to your right where the Chapel is."

There is also a small pharmacy.

Weinberg 5—the wing Gary was on—had thirty-four rooms. By the time Gary left the hospital, he had been in eight of them.

Carol trusted Gary's main team: Dr. Jonathan Chun, Dr. Luther Holton III, and Dr. Raymond Cross Jr.

Dr. Chun—a specialist in colon and rectal surgery—was going to reconstruct Gary's intestines and to take down the ileostomy—a loop of the small intestine connected to the surface of the skin—and remove his gall bladder. Doctor Luther Holton III—a Temple University School of Medicine trained plastic surgeon, who treats everything from benign tumors to burn injuries, from skin cancer to gastrointestinal diseases—would do reconstruction surgery on Gary.

"I love that man," Carol said about Dr. Chun.

Dr. Cross was a gastroenterology specialist who had graduated from the University of Pittsburg School of Medicine in 1997.

"[W]hen [Gary] came to us, he was quite ill," Dr. Cross said, "and . . . he had a number of surgical complications that probably were misdiagnosed . . . [H]e was a mess."

Dr. Chun found Gary irritable and difficult to work with. But Carol was always there, and "was consistent; she was amazingly resilient throughout this process in being a go-between our doctors, and between him . . . [S]he never waver[ed]."

Dr. Chun found it hard to explain why it was so hard to close Gary up.

"[B]asically," Dr. Chun said, Gary "had a hostile abdomen, so he had had multiple procedures, and so there's going to be tons of scar tissue, you have all these inflammatory tracts throughout, connecting intestine to loops of bowel, and it was just . . . a difficult operation . . . [Y]ou're trying to save as much intestines as you can, because if you take too much out, then you're not going to be able to use your intestinal tract, and you're going to be dependent on nutrition through the vein to survive. So, our surgeons were trying to . . . repair these areas, and save as much bowel as possible, and for whatever reason, you know, these fistulas came back, and all these areas . . . [were] open . . ."

"We could not control his pain," Dr. Chun said. "[H]is pain was so terrible, he was requiring so much pain medicine, and it wasn't something really that was easily reversible . . . [H]e wasn't able to be discharged."

An ostomy is an artificial opening in the body. Gary had so many ostomy appliances "over these fistulas to collect the liquid," Dr. Chun said, " . . . it was a mess."

But Carol wasn't giving up.

Chun said he had never met a woman with Carol's indomitable will. It was clear how much Gary and Carol loved each other.

# 27

"[W]hen people get sick," Dr. Chun explained, ". . . they have all kinds of different reactions . . ."

It can bring out the best in people, and sometimes, Dr. Chun said, "it brings out the very worst in people. . . [A]t times, it brought out the worst in Gary, and I think if I had known Gary before all this, he probably would have been quite different. I think once he was better, he was clearly a different person."

Dr. Chun didn't know Carol before he met Gary.

"I think she's an example of an extreme," Dr. Chun said, "you know, the top 10 or 15 percent of people that are amazingly resilient under enormous stress, and . . . [making] decisions that place an incredible burden on her. And I think that she was remarkably resilient."

However, Carol's support did not guarantee Gary's survival. Dr. Chun thought that Gary's "odds of surviving were very, very low. Certainly, he was going to succumb to some kind of infection, or overdose of narcotics, or aspiration pneumonia, or something would have happened to him. His long-term prognosis was . . . bleak . . ."

# 28

---

"Things started going really fast," Carol said. "Dr. Cross testing, Dr. Chun testing, infectious disease testing, dietitian, and Joan the wound nurse helping me with Gary's open abdomen."

Dr. Cross told Carol that Gary had no active Crohn's, and he didn't think Gary was going to survive.

"It was as if a light went off in his head," Carol said. "He stared out into space, then looked at me and said what about a fungi cocktail?"

Fungi?

Carol had visions of Gary on peyote. Another Happy Place for Gary to go to?

The fungi cocktail was an anti-viral drug.

I bet Gary has a fungal infection, the doctor said. He decided to give Gary a twenty-one-day IV infusion.

Carol agreed. No one had tried that.

Don't let him have Prednisone, Dr. Cross said. Don't let him have Toradol ever again.

"And I was like, oh, my God, they knew what they were doing," Carol said.

Not only does this man never get Prednisone again, Dr. Cross said, but any time a doctor tries to give it to him, you are to tell him he's allergic to it.

"Gary and I had been at the University of Maryland for a month or so," Carol said, "when his numbers were down, his infections were gone, he was alert."

But his body had been mutilated, his stomach was wide open, and he had a central line for TPN—liquid nutrition—and pain medication.

"Have you named it yet?" Joan the wound nurse asked.

"It?" Gary asked.

"Your fistula," Joan said. "People name them."

"Hermie," Gary said. " Hermie."

While Gary was open, Hermie sometimes emerged, swelling, almost upright like the monster who attacks the crew in "Alien."

"Dr. Chun laughed his butt off when he found out I called it that," Gary would later say.

When Dr. Chun laughed, his eyes would close. Gary did a good imitation.

Dr. Chun said that he was going to have to take Hermie out, but he was not going to do it until he was ready to close Gary up.

Carol liked all of Gary's doctors at the Univeristy of Maryland, but she knew that "Dr. Chun took Gary and me home with him every night. It's what he thought of when [he] went to bed, it's what he and his wife talked about during dinner, and he was trying to get all these other people involved to find out what was going on in Gary, because he was supposed to close Gary up in January."

# 29

Things were going better at the University of Maryland Hospital. It was Saturday. Stacey was going to visit.

"Are you feeling well enough to get cleaned up?" Carol asked Gary.

"I would love a shave," Gary said.

"Oh, wow," Carol said, "you really want to get cleaned up! You must be feeling better?"

"Yes," Gary said. "I am."

Carol called David and asked him to bring Gary's razor and shaving supplies, shower soap, shampoo, and conditioner.

"And deodorant," Gary called out.

"And deodorant," Carol added. "Have you let the dogs out?"

"I'm on my way to the house now," David said. "I'll see you in about an hour."

Carol ended the call. "Do you want a sponge bath?" Carol asked Gary.

"I want to get into the shower," Gary said. Another good sign, Carol figured.

Carol came around the bed to help Gary stand.

"Are you really up to this?" Carol asked.

"I need it," Gary said.

"Then," Carol said, "that's what we'll do." Carol went to the nurses' station and told Gary's nurse the plan.

"I need something to put over Gary's stomach because he is going to take a shower," Carol said. "When he gets out, can you change his central line dressing?"

The nurse said <u>Sure,</u> and asked if Carol needed help getting Gary into the shower.

"I need you to give Gary his pain medicine now," Carol said. "And then again when he gets out of the shower."

<u>You sure you don't want my help giving him the shower?</u> the nurse asked.

"Gary's brother and sister in-law will help me," Carol said.

<u>Okay,</u> the nurse said. <u>I'll get you everything you need.</u>

"And a shower chair," Carol said. Back in Gary's room, Carol told Gary, "We're getting everything ready. The nurse'll give you some pain meds. "

"Okay," Gary said. "Let's start now."

"We need to wait for David," Carol said.

"We can start with flushing out my bag," Gary said.

"I can do that," Carol said.

She long ago had gotten used to the creature part of Gary's illness. And, even faced with an unusual mess, Carol kept her vow never to let Gary see her feel any disgust with anything having to do with him.

"No," Gary said. "I want to do it. I want to learn how." Carol showed him. Gary's need for independence was yet another good sign.

David came in.

"What's up?" David asked.

"Gary is having a good day," Carol said. "He wants to shave."

"I brought everything you need," David said. "And I stopped and picked up a mirror."

David arranged everything so Gary could shave in bed. David held the mirror. As Gary shaved, he sang an old Yiddish song.

Stacey entered and asked, "What's going on?"

"The three of us are going to give Gary a shower," Carol said.

"What?" Stacey asked.

"Gary wants to have a shower," Carol said, "so I thought we would all help him."

Gary, Stacey, and David all laughed.

"Um, okay," David said.

"We can do that," Stacey said. "Let's do it," Gary said.

Gary hadn't seemed this energetic and engaged for a long time.

The nurse came in with more toiletries and equipment Gary might need. It took them twenty minutes to maneuver Gary into the shower.

"Okay," Stacey said, "I'll step out for a minute."

"You're getting in here with me," Gary said.

Carol and David covered Gary stomach with a plastic bag and took off his gown.

"Okay, Stacey," Gary said. "You can get in the shower with me."

"Let's do this," Stacey said, climbing into the shower. Nothing phased her. She was a nurse. "Everything you see," she said later, "is just another body part."

Carol wore shorts and a tank top. David wore shorts and a shirt. Stacey had on a nice pair of slacks and a nice blouse.

"I'm not dressed for this," she said.

"Don't you mean you are dressed for this," Gary said.

Carol adjusted the water so it was warm.

She was behind Gary. David was on the right side, Stacey was on the left side. The detachable shower head had a long line. Carol got Gary's hair wet and handed the shower head to David—the wrong way. Soaking him.

"Oops," Carol said. "Sorry."

All four were in hysterics.

"Stacey," Carol gasped in between laughing, "can you hand me the shampoo?"

"I'm getting cold," Gary said.

"I'm getting wet," Stacey said.

David rinsed the shampoo from Gary's hair.

"Stacey," Carol said, "hand me the conditioner."

David continued to rinse Gary's hair. The water fell over Gary's face in sheets.

"I should of taken my top off," David said.

"I should of taken my shoes off," Stacey said.

Carol looked down at her soaked self and said, "Me, too."

"Okay," Stacey said, "we are laughing too much."

"Everyone going by this room I'm sure is wondering what's going on in here," David said.

"Who cares," Gary said. "This is the best I've felt in months."

"David, Stacey, and I wanted to laugh and cry at the same time," Carol said.

# 30

September 4, 2011. The Grand Prix was going to be held in downtown Baltimore, which had never happened before. The race track was one block from the hospital. The cars had been practicing for a few days. Gary could hear them from his hospital room.

"A few years earlier, Gary had driven a NASCAR," Carol said, "and was black-flagged for going too fast."

David and Stacey had come down to the hospital.

"What's going on?" he asked. Innocently.

"I'm ready to get out of here," Gary said.

"Gary's having a good day," Carol explained.

"You don't want to leave now," Stacey said. "It's crazy outside with the race cars and the traffic."

"It took us an hour to find a parking spot," David said.

"We've been listening to them practice for days," Carol said.

"What time does the racing start?" Gary asked. Not so innocent.

Carol, David, and Stacey exchanged glances.

"I'm not sure," David said. "I think it starts at 10 or 11."

"I wish I could see it," Gary said, studying them.

They all grinned.

"I'll be right back," Carol said.

She walked into the hall. Stacey followed her.

"You heard Gary," Carol said. "He wants to go to the races."

Taking Gary outside was, of course, against hospital policy.

"How are we going to do this?" Stacey asked.

"I'm going to make sure that Sparky"—the security guard—"is downstairs so we can get out. Get a wheelchair. I'll let Gary's nurse know we are taking Gary for a walk."

"What if she asks if we are planning to take him outside?" Stacey asked.

"I'll ask him if he's seen it outside," Carol said. "I'll tell him it's crazy outside, and that we would have to be crazy to take him out there."

"Okay," Stacey said, "well, maybe we shouldn't. It *is* a little crazy out there."

"There are three of us." Carol said, "and you're the best nurse ever. And, if you don't believe me, ask Gary. He tells everyone that."

"What do you need me to do?" Stacey asked.

"Give me ten minutes," Carol said. "As soon as I know Sparky is downstairs, I will send you a text. Then you and David start getting Gary ready."

Carol went downstairs. Sparky was at the side door. Carol grabbed a wheelchair, casually said hi to Sparky, took the wheelchair upstairs, and went up to Gary's nurse.

"I have a question," Carol said. "Is it almost time for Gary's medication?"

I have it right here, she said.

"Good," Carol said. "His brother is here. We're taking Gary out of the room for a while."

How long are you going to be gone? the nurse asked.

"When Gary starts getting tired," Carol said, "which shouldn't be too long."

Do you need my help?

"Only to give Gary his medication."

When Carol got back into the room, Gary was all set to go. The nurse followed and gave Gary his meds.

Have a good walk, Mr. Stern, the nurse said. Then she walked out.

"What are you up to?" Gary asked.

"Just taking you for a walk," Carol said, "and getting you out of this room."

The four of them got into the elevator.

"Okay," Gary said, "now, what's going on?"

"We're going to see the race," David said.

Followed by David and Stacey, Carol pushed Gary in his wheelchair to the side door.

"Hey, Sparky," Carol said. "We're going to the races."

Have a good time, Sparky said.

It was sunny, about 80°F. A great day for the race. David pushed Gary in the wheelchair. Carol and Stacey strolled along beside. They found the perfect spot at one of the restaurants. The cars were so loud that the vibrations shook the table—and Gary's chair.

"Gary looked as if he were back in his NASCAR, getting black-flagged all over again," Carol said. "For the next hour, the four of us just hung out, having fun."

# 31

Dr. Chun wanted Gary to heal enough and get strong enough to survive the surgery. To recuperate, Gary needed to:

1. only have four ounces of water a day
2. stay open with the fistula bag
3. live on TPN (liquid nutrition)

"Oh, yes, and number four, go to a rehab," some doctors were suggesting.

"Excuse me?" Carol said. "Rehab?"

A halfway house.

It's been more than twenty-one days, Dr. Chun said, his white count is normal, and we've got his lipids where they should be.

"Over my dead body," Carol said.

Carol, Dr. Chun said, you don't have a choice. You don't have insurance. We've got things under control. Gary is going to be coming back here to have surgery to get closed up, but he needs to go someplace else, and you can't take him home because no company that deals with TPN and the other supplies—particularly pain-killers—is going to take him without insurance.

"Dr. Chun," Carol said, "I guess you don't know me very well yet. You've seen what I can do with medical records and taking care of my husband. Let me show you what I can really do. My husband's not going to a halfway house. He's going home with me, and I'm going to take care of him. Give me twenty-four hours."

Carol barged into the case manager's office.

"I cried," Carol said. "I got mad, and I cried some more."

She told the case manager she wasn't even going to tell Gary how awful the place was that they had recommended. And she said, "I'm taking [Gary] home." That night she prayed. And she prayed the next morning, September 7, which was Gary's birthday.

Dr. Chun came in and told Gary he was being moved that day to the rehab. Gary started crying. Carol caught up with Dr. Chun in the hall and asked him to give her a few more hours, which he said he would.

Carol went back into the room, where Gary was still crying.

"I'm not going to let you down," Carol said.

"I was telling myself that, too," Carol said.

She took Gary's hand. She wiped the tears from his face and told him not to worry. She would be taking him home.

Gary asked how she was going to manage that.

"I told him I was going to take care of it," Carol said.

She walked out of Gary's room, praying as hard as she could.

"I started to go up to the nurses' station," Carol said, "when I heard someone call my name from behind me.

Miss Stern, Miss Stern.

The case manager was hurrying after Carol. She had a lady with her who wore "a suit with a monogram on its chest," Carol said.

The woman with the monogram introduced herself as Kim from Equinox Services, the company that would be providing TPN and other medications to Gary at home.

If Carol could get him home.

"After two hours of phone calls and conversations and giving my word I would make sure they were paid," Carol said—a promise Carol kept. Carol thought they had made some progress.

"Kim talked to the owner of the company," Carol said, " and told him I had given my word that I would do everything in my power to get my husband Medicare and Medicaid as quickly as possible, so I could have him home and he could have what he needed."

Equinox gambled on Carol's certainty.

"I was sitting in the room with Gary," Carol said, "and I got a text on my phone to please come to the nurses' station."

Kim took Carol into an office.

"She took a deep breath and smiled," Carol said.

She had arranged for her company to make sure Gary had what he needed.

"She told me not to worry about it," Carol said.

Again, Carol started crying.

"I told her it was Gary's birthday," Carol said. "She said, 'Go give him his birthday present.' I said, 'No, you're the one that made this happen, so you should give it to him.'"

Together they went into Gary's room. Carol introduced Kim, who said, I heard it was your birthday today.

"Yes," Gary said. "It is."

I have a present for you, Kim said.

"Ya?" Gary said.

Happy birthday. You're not going to rehab. You're going home.

"I don't understand," Gary said.

He knew they didn't have the money to cover the expenses involved in Gary going home.

My company, Equinox, is going to supply your TPN and any other IV meds you need, Kim said.

"Really," Gary said. "Really?"

Gary started crying. Kim started crying. Carol was already crying.

On September 7, 2011, Gary's forty-eighth birthday, he would be discharged. He'd take his TPN, liquid nutrition, at home.

## 32

Right before Gary was discharged, Dr. Chun had a meeting with him, Carol, and David and explained that Gary needed bowel rest. No foods passing through his system.

"For how long this time?" David asked.

Dr. Chun said he wasn't sure. Gary had to stay on TPN and NPO—nil per os (nothing by mouth)—for at least three more months.

Shakily, and Gary rarely sounded so shaky, Gary said, Not three months."

"It'll be okay," Carol said.

"Then, what?" Gary asked.

The doctors tended to think in immediate terms: How can he hold on until the next day. Gary thought in long-range terms: How can I survive what I'm going through.

Dr. Chun said he would take Gary off the TPN and NPO when Gary was healed and without fistulas. Then, Gary would get his belly reconstructed.

"No," Gary said. "Not a skin graft."

"I have plenty of skin," David said. "They can take mine."

# 33

---

Angela Mason became Gary and Carol's Equinox ongoing contact. People who have never used TPN would ask Mason what she did.

"What do I tell them?" Mason asked. "[I]f I tell them I'm [a] dietician, they usually say, 'Oh, so you can tell me what to eat.' And I say, I don't take care of patients that eat, if my patients are eating . . . [they] don't need my services, and they get this glaze look and ask again . . . 'what do you do?'"

When people learn they have to be on TPN, they "are completely stunned because something has gone terribly, terribly wrong in [their] life."

Mason explained "It's always a tough thing at the beginning. It's very overwhelming. All of a sudden, [your home] . . . looks like a hospital room with all sorts of IV bags in the home setting, and this is not what most people sign up for. . . [I]t's a life-changer. It is completely life-altering, especially with folks who never, who are not able to continue to eat. . . [I]t's life-altering for both the person who needs the parenteral nutrition and the family."

The patients Mason handled often used the liquid nutrition for bowel rest, "especially," Mason said, "if the fistulas are large and if there's a lot coming out of them. Bowel rest means that you are resting the intestinal tract. So you are not eating or drinking, or if you are, it's very, very minimal amounts of maybe like ice chips, water, clear liquids. And parenteral nutrition is IV nutrition. It's a sterile solution of amino acids, dextrose, intravenous lipids, electrolytes, multivitamins, trace elements. Calories, protein, hydration, monitoring his lab work, making sure that he didn't have any electrolyte abnormalities. Because this bypasses the GI tract, it can create some significant problems with the liver, which Gary eventually developed: Parenteral nutrition is associated with liver disease, so we had to make some modifications to his nutrition based on that."

Gary got his TPN over a twelve-hour period. They couldn't run it twenty-four hours a day, because it would overwhelm the liver.

"If you have too many calories," Mason said, "you develop a fatty liver," – which could cause cirrhosis and scarring. "We had to restrict the amount of lipids that we were providing him."

Mason thought Gary "was . . . pretty good looking" even though "he was . . . very debilitated. . . He seemed like a really nice guy to me. Carol was a little bit of a surprise. She was not how I had envisioned her. You spend a lot of time talking to people over the phone and you sort of develop this picture in your mind about them, and Carol was not what I had expected for some reason."

Mason had pictured Carol as "taller and with darker hair."

Gary and Carol were "so appreciative and so thankful for the care that I had been providing, and the company had been providing. I also got to take a look at some of Gary's wounds, and his fistulas, and those were pretty dramatic. I spent a lot of time working in hospitals, including trauma centers, and I've seen a lot of gnarly, gnarly wounds, and his were pretty big, his were pretty dramatic. So I was pretty impressed with the fact that Carol had been able to [take care of them] . . . Most folks would not have been able to manage somebody that medically complex at home, and Carol did it single-handedly for the most part."

But "Carol was anxious, very, very anxious," Mason said, "which is not uncommon. Most people have never heard of parenteral nutrition, and then all of a sudden you're now being told that you have to do this very complex medical therapy for your loved one at home, and it's usually something pretty calamitous if you do require parenteral nutrition. It's frequently something very calamitous, which in Gary's case it was."

Mason thought Carol was "very, very proficient at caring for Gary, with all of his medical aspects, but she would sometimes lose the forest for the trees."

Carol—Mason thought—was hypervigilant about everything that went on with him.

"She created a lot of anxiety for herself," Mason said "because of that hypervigilance. Having said that, her vigilance probably saved [Gary] from further complications, such as infections, and so forth and so on, but she was very, very stressed in taking care of him."

Mason "never expected Gary's fistulas to heal up . . . [A]s soon as one started to heal up, he would pop another one."

Mason focused on trying to prevent any "life-threatening infection."

Life-threatening infections are common for patients on chronic parenteral nutrition, "because," Mason said, "you are developing, you're infusing a very nutrient-rich formula into your central venous system, and bacteria love that formula, which is why you need to do it under sterile techniques."

Carol told Mason that they were having financial problems.

Home infusion of TPN is not inexpensive, over one hundred dollars a day.

"And Gary was having problems with his insurance," Mason said, " . . . going between Medicare and Medicaid and so forth and so on, medical assistance."

Equinox—Mason explained—is "a for profit company. [W]e can't always do charity cases, because if we did that, then we wouldn't be able to take care of anyone. But, yeah, I . . . plugged their case . . . [T]here was a financial decision, but there was also . . . an emotional decision . . . Gary had gone through so much . . . [I]t wasn't . . . his fault that he was in the position that he was in. And there was Carol, who was . . . struggling and working so hard, and doing everything that she could to . . . care for Gary."

More than 40,000 people in America are solely dependent on TPN to survive.

The CEO of the company decided that "we were not going to simply abandon Gary and Carol just because their insurance was in limbo," Mason said. "We knew that that was going to eventually be resolved . . . and we would eventually write off the cost of it."

Very unusual.

"[W]e knew that this was going to be a lifelong thing for Carol and Gary," Mason said. "[W]e were never going to recoup what we lost . . ."

# 34

Carol took Gary home.

David met them at the house; but, when they got there, there was no electricity.

"My electricity bill was paid," Carol said, "so I thought maybe somebody had hit a pole."

One more thing to contend with. Carol worried that Gary would stress over it. An hour later, the power came on. A nurse from Equinox—from which they were getting the TPN—showed up with all the supplies.

David stayed most of the night.

The three of them sat in the living room.

September 11, 2011.

They were home for three days. Gary was feeling good; but, after a while, he said he wasn't feeling right.

It didn't seem urgent. Carol went upstairs to take a quick shower. When she came back down, Butchy wasn't barking. He howled in—Carol said—"a screeching tone."

Gary was sprawled out "like a board." The fistula bag had broken. Gary was turning blue around the mouth and choking on his own saliva.

"I ran to the front door," Carol said, "and yelled to any neighbor" who might be around, "Call 911."

"What's wrong?" her next-door neighbors asked.

"Just call 911," Carol said.

The neighbors, renters who had just moved into 8008 Green Valley Lane, had come to Gary and Carol's defense when they were under fire from the homeowners' association, which didn't like their Christmas lights.

"The homeowners' association were just rude, obnoxious, Carol said. "Once they heard what happened with Gary, they changed very quickly."

The homeowners told the association to leave the Sterns alone.

Gary had had a seizure. He went limp and had aspirated vomit. Carol started mouth to mouth on Gary.

She could hear the ambulance siren approaching as Gary started coming around.

While they were wheeling Gary to the ambulance, he was in what Carol called "his happy place."

As usual, whenever Gary came out of a Grand Mal seizure, he would see flowers and he would talk very low and he would say he could see a glow around Carol.

"What's all the lights around you?" he once asked.

And then he would come out of it.

"Sometimes Gary's post-seizure calm would last a couple of minutes, sometimes it would last up to twenty minutes," Carol said. "It depends on how bad the seizures were."

The ambulance took Gary to the nearest hospital. The choice was either Sinai or Northwest. Carol did _not_ want to go back to Sinai.

"We had gone to the other hospital, University," Carol said. "They had gotten everything under control. But University Hospital was too far away."

Carol called David and Barbara, who met them at the Northwest ER, where Gary had another seizure.

After running tests, the doctors told Carol that Gary's seizures were a result of withdrawal from Benzodiazepine, which they had been giving Gary in the hospital.

"Giving him a lot of it," Carol said—and giving it for so long his body had gotten used to it.

"When Gary had been sent home," Carol said, "one of the doctors didn't give me the script for the liquid Ativan, which is a benzodiazepine."

The seizure was likely a result of Gary stopping the drug. The Ativan might have prevented Gary from having a seizure.

"Where the hell is his Ativan?" Carol said in the hospital. "Give this man two milligrams of Ativan. I don't care if the doctors ordered it or not, just give it to him."

If he aspirated, the doctors would have to intubate him. Carol didn't want that. They took Gary up to the third floor, which was an IMC unit, a step down from the ICU. The nurses there knew Carol.

"I promised that I wouldn't give their names," if they gave Gary the Ativan, Carol said.

Several medical personnel there told Carol that she needed to get Gary's records from his hospitals.

"I already have them," Carol said.

Carol refused to sign discharge papers for Gary until they gave Gary a hospital bed for home—which insurance did not cover.

"What is it going to take to get you to sign these papers," the case manager asked. " What if I promise you that the hospital [will deliver the bed] . . . within two hours?"

"Well, then," Carol said, "we'll be leaving in two and a half hours."

"Seriously," the case nurse said, "this is what it's going to take?"

"It's either that," Carol said, "or I have every newscast, news media down here within the next thirty-five minutes, and if you don't think it's possible, try me."

Carol told the case nurse she had the hospital records.

"Do you want to do it this way," delivering the hospital bed to their home, "or do you want to do it with an attorney, and the news media?"

At home, Gary had been sleeping on an air mattress.

The case manager told Carol it was . . . possible.

"Make it possible tomorrow," Carol said.

The next day, David went to the house.

"The bed is set up," he called Carol, "and Stacey has made the bed."

"Does it work?" Carol asked.

"Yes," he said.

The next day, Gary walked out of the hospital.

Before Gary left, the nurses, PAs, and some doctors at Northwest all wanted to know how Gary was doing. When Carol told them, a few would say, I'm sorry, and some would say I hope he gets better. A few just looked down, guiltily.

"They knew something, no one was telling me," Carol said.

One or two of those who had looked down sought Carol out and told her she needed to look into this, but they weren't specific about what this was.

One told her to get an attorney.

# 35

"After we first got Gary home from the hospital," Carol said, "we had gone to see an attorney, Steven Snyder, the second-best malpractice lawyer in Maryland.

"They said because Gary's had Crohn's his whole life, it would be a hard case to prove," David said. "My father was friends with Snyder." Which is why they went to him first. "His kids are attorneys" in the same practice. "When he got wind that his kids had turned our case down, you can believe he gave his kids a hard time."

"A very hard time," Carol said.

"Gary, Carol, and I all knew there was problems," David said. "It seemed to us like negligence, but we weren't thinking like that, we were just thinking to get him better, and then down the road, if there's anything to look into, we'll look into. That's all we were thinking about, trying to get Gary better."

Carol listed the "Things I needed to know, check, and do for Gary."

Another list of things to take care of once Gary was home included how to keep the central line clean, so Gary wouldn't develop infections, and how to change Gary's line-dressing once a week.

TPN has a lot of sugar, which could cause diabetes. TPN doesn't have vitamin D or iron. TPN may have lipids (fat). TPN might not be enough to keep Gary hydrated. Every week the TPN had to be adjusted depending on Gary's blood work. TPN has to be refrigerated until used.

Once taken out of the refrigerator, Carol had to wait until the TPN was at room temperature before adding supplements.

After infusing the TPN with supplements, the TPN had to be started within three hours. And TPN is only good for twenty-four hours. An hour after she started infusion, Carol had to check Gary's blood every four hours until the TPN stopped.

Long term, TPN will cause kidney failure and liver damage. Carol struggled with that knowledge that every day she was giving Gary TPN to keep him alive.

"But I was also killing him," Carol said.

# 36

Carol put three books together. One: Gary's doctors and phone numbers, appointments, and his medication list. Two: Gary's vitals. And three: Gary's ER book with everything the ER doctor might need from them.

All Gary's medication was liquid form and there was a lot of medication. Carol organized color-coded syringes. She color-coded the medication bottles. She wrote down when and how much Gary would take of each substance.

But Carol had other things to do, like find money to pay their expenses. Gary's fistula bags cost over $300 for six, and his medication was hundreds and hundreds of dollars each week. The bank continued to threaten to foreclose on the house.

"People were coming over to see Gary," Carol said, "making me out to be the bad guy because I wouldn't let Gary have a sip of water."

Gary would say he was parched.

"Gary loved the word parched," Carol said. "I think he said it to piss me off."

The visitors would look at Carol and say, "Oh, give him a drink. How could one drink hurt?"

One drink could kill him.

Carol told the visitors to stop hassling her or to get out.

## 37

Carol had started preparing the paperwork for Medicaid right after Gary went into Northwest. The day after Gary was released from Northwest, on September 12, 2011, Carol got a letter from the Social Security Administration. She was excited. The letter must mean that Gary had been declared disabled, so they were going to get help paying Gary's medical bills. She didn't want to open the letter on her own. She ran into the house and gave the letter to Gary, who handed it back to her.

"Open it," he said.

Carol did. And started reading out loud: "We are sorry to inform you that we cannot deem you disabled at this time."

"What?" Carol said. "I got a flashback of everything Gary had been through for the last five months. I looked at Gary, and my heart—Oh, my heart started to break."

But her inner voice told Carol, *Keep it together. Don't let Gary see you upset.*

"Babe," Carol told Gary, "don't you worry about this. I was told you always get denied the first time."

She sent David a text: *Can you come over? I need to make a call.* David knew what she meant was that she needed to do something without upsetting Gary.

Carol contacted Governor O'Malley's office, where she spoke to the woman in charge of disability, Anne. Carol faxed her a signed consent form, allowing the office to ask about Gary's case. About two days later, Anne called Carol to let her know she had the fax and would get back to her the beginning of the following week.

"My husband doesn't have that much time," Carol said. "Do you have a strong stomach?"

Carol kept her on the line and told her about what happened to Gary and what kind of condition he was in and their financial situation.

"His abdomen is open," Carol said. "His intestines are on the outside of his stomach."

Anne assured Carol she would do everything she could to help.

A few hours later, Anne called back and said I've been thinking about you and Gary ever since we got off the phone. I'm going to work really hard to help you two.

Anne told Carol she had arranged for an emergency interview with Social Security over the phone at two o'clock the next day.

On the phone, Carol began: "I received a letter stating my husband was denied disability. Can you tell me why?"

SS: Let me see. I see your husband's case has been red flagged.

Carol: "What does that mean?"

SS: That means someone has been inquiring about the case.

Carol: "Such as the Governor's Office?"

SS: Yes.

Was Carol being punished for pressing her case?

Carol: "Okay. I know about him. What else does it say?"

SS: The only thing I see is at this time is are doctors do not believe Mr. Stern is disabled.

Carol went bat-shit.

Carol: "What? My husband isn't disabled? I'm looking at my husband in a hospital bed in my home. His intestines are on the outside of his stomach. He only gets medicine and nutrition through an IV line. He can barely talk on the phone. And your doctors are stating that my husband is not disabled? Why don't you tell them to come over here and look at him and tell <u>me</u>."

SS: <u>Well, Mrs. Stern, you have the right to appeal.</u>

Carol: "And how long will that take?"

SS: <u>About eighteen months to twenty-four months.</u>

Carol: "You have got to be kidding. My husband doesn't have that kind of time!"

SS: <u>There's nothing I can do.</u>

Carol: "Maybe *you* can't but I will find someone who can."

Carol got off the phone. "I was so mad I went back into the house and looked at Gary," Carol said.

"Not disabled?"

Seeing Carol's expression, Gary said, "What now?"

As usual, trying to protect Gary from bad news, Carol dismissed the phone call.

"Just a lot of BS," she said. "Nothing I can't take care of."

Carol could take pictures of Gary to show them, to prove that Gary was, in fact, disabled. Which she did. The photographs show Gary's entrails open to the air.

"People don't understand what I'm talking about until I show them the pictures of Gary's open abdomen," Carol said. "It's like Jackie Kennedy said when she refused to change out of the blood-stained clothes she was wearing: when the President was assassinated' I want them to see what they've done to him.'"

"Babe," Carol said, "I'm going to take another picture," which she did, of Gary's intestines.

She emailed it to the Obamas, saying, "Please, call me," and included her phone number.

No one responded.

# 38

Carol hired Fred London, a lawyer who specialized in Disability Insurance.

London's office explained to Carol that Social Security Disability Insurance depends on medical records. You have to prove the recipient has been disabled for over a year. Social Security Insurance—not the Disability Insurance—is needs-based. You don't have to have worked for a year, but you do have to supply income and assets to prove financial hardships, a harder process.

Carol arranged their house in Owings Mills so it looked like a hospital room.

She called London's office and was told it was going to take another eight months before they could get a decision on Gary's disability.

Carol had so many things going through her head: no money, no insurance, Gary needed medication and TPN.

Carol made a promise to Equinox (where she got her TPN) that she would be able to cover the cost of the nutrition.

She was overwhelmed and began to fear they could not make it.

"Then I heard that voice," Carol said. *Don't give up now. You can do this.*

One of her angels.

## 39

About ten the next morning, Anne called from the Governor's office.

I . . . just got off the phone, I got a call from the senator's office—the State Senator, Anne said. How is your husband doing today?

"He has good moments and bad moments," Carol said. "Thank you for asking."

And how are you doing today? Anne asked.

"That depends on what you tell me," Carol said.

I spoke to Mr. Cardin—Maryland Senator Benjamin Cardin—yesterday afternoon, he told me to make your husband top priority.

"That's great."

That's the good news.

"And the bad?"

In order to be eligible for Medicare you have to be declared disabled by the government, which the government couldn't do, Carol was told, because Gary's last official work date was seven months earlier, which means Gary's chance to get Medicare has expired.

"Let me get this straight. To get state help, the federal government has to say it's okay?"

We don't put it like that . . .

"It really doesn't matter how you put it," Carol said. Crying (and Carol hated how much she had been crying lately), Carol said, "He doesn't have time."

We understand that . . . Do you have an attorney?

"Fred London," Carol said.

I am going to contact them, Anne said, and let them know we will be helping you.

Anne said their office was also going to ask for an emergency hearing in front of a judge.

It's going to take about two weeks before you go in front of the judge, Ann told Carol.

"Okay," Carol said.

Then, came the questions, about Gary's doctors, letters with Gary's diagnosis. Anne wanted to know if anything showed that Gary was disabled. She asked Carol to fax what she had.

"Right away," Carol said.

Anne also asked for a photo of Gary, which struck Carol as promising. Anne wanted to make Gary an individual, with a face, not merely a case.

She told Carol not to fax the photos of Gary since he was sick. Not yet. Do you think your husband can get in front of the Judge?

"Absolutely not," Carol said.

Carol explained she had Gary's power of attorney.

That will work, Anne said. I'm going to get all of this started. You fax me the papers from the doctor, and I will call you when we have a court date.

Carol, who had been talking to Anne while on the porch, went into the house and told Gary what was going on. Gary started to cry.

"It's my job to take care of you," Gary said, "not your job to take care of me."

Carol sat at the edge of the bed and wiped Gary's tears. She took his hand.

"You've been taking care of us and me for years," she said. "Let me take care of us."

Gary squeezed Carol's hand.

"We have always been 50/50," Carol reminded him.

"50/50," Gary said.

# 40

---

"I have all your medical records," Carol told Gary before their court date. "I didn't tell you. When you first got to University, the doctors were asking for your medical records.

She called Sinai but felt they were giving her the runaround. Finally, Carol got the records herself, by calling in a favor from the head of the hospital whom she had met in the elevator.

# 41

---

A few days later Theresa, one of the lawyer's assistants, called Carol.

I spoke to an assistant from Senator Cardin's office. She said she was going to help us with Mr. Stern's case.

"Yes," Carol said. "I called the Senator's office a few days ago."

Wow, Theresa said, "you don't mess around.

"And I don't take no for an answer," Carol said.

We have a date with the judge on November 3, Theresa said. "At 10:00 a.m."

"I was hoping it would be in October," Carol said.

This was the first available date, Theresa said, but don't worry. I need you to put all of Mr. Stern's medical receipts together.

"All?"

Medication, supplies, doctors' bills, hospital bills.

"Do you have any idea how many hospital bills I have? They started coming days after Gary first went into the hospital. I get three or four piles a week."

"Great."

"Not great," Carol said. "I don't have the money to pay them."

I didn't mean that, Theresa said. I meant we can show how much help you need.

A few hours later, an assistant from Senator Cardin's office called Carol. She had been going over the same information that Theresa had been looking at. The only difference was that she told Carol she was going to call at least once a week—which she did—and she gave Carol her cell phone number and told Carol she could call her day or night.

It took Carol two weeks to arrange the medical and financial records, everything, in a binder.

"You can get anything done," Gary told her—and laughed so hard that Hermie popped out.

Once, when he asked Carol what she was doing in the kitchen, Carol said, "Right now, I'm sending a picture of Hermie."

Gary laughed harder.

"There's nothing you're not going to do for me," he said, "is there?"

"Babe," Carol said, "if I could cut my stomach open and lay in that bed for you, I would do it."

Theresa from Gary's lawyer's office called her the day before the court date.

I wanted to let you know that I'll be at the court house at 10:15, Theresa said.

"But court starts at 10."

If they call the case before I get there, Theresa said, just tell them we are going to ask for a continuance.

Continuance? Carol thought. Kiss my ass.

"Why?" she asked.

I don't have everything together for what we need.

"Well," Carol said, "I do. I'm ready for this." Maybe I should meet you at 9:30, then.

# 42

November 3, 2011, Kenny, David, and Stacey stayed with Gary. Carol put on a dark blue suit, checked her briefcase, which had all her paperwork. She had made four copies of everything: one for the judge, one for Gary's attorney, one for the state attorney, and one for herself.

Outside, the building looked like a regular courthouse. Inside, it looked more like a Social Security or a DMV office.

It was 9:30, and Carol wasn't sure what to do or where to go.

"I'm here for my husband," Carol told a security guard. "Gary Stern."

Behind her, someone said, Mrs. Stern?

Carol turned around and saw a woman who looked like she was still in high school. She had long dark hair, black slacks, and a gray sweater that looked like it was two sizes too big.

"Please, please," Carol thought, "don't be from Gary's attorney's office."

The woman in the too big sweater said she was Theresa from Fred London's office.

Carol thought, "We're screwed."

Theresa suggested they go into a corner and talk.

I need to make sure you understand that the chance of getting a judgment in our favor is slim to none, Theresa said. Maybe 1 to 2 percent.

"Okay," Carol said. "We'll be that one percent."

Carol unsnapped her briefcase and took out her color-coded folders.

"The red one is for the judge," Carol said.

Theresa went over Carol's papers.

When Mr. Stern's case is called, let me do the talking, Theresa said.

"Sure," Carol said, thinking, Yeah, I'm going to let you do the talking. Not.

The courtroom struck Carol more like a conference room than a court. There was a long table. At the far end sat a woman dressed in a suit, the judge.

The meeting lasted about forty minutes. Carol did 90 percent of the talking, "which," Carol said, "as you can tell, I'm really good at doing."

Carol couldn't stop thinking about how young Theresa was.

"They've got a state attorney," Carol thought. "And I've got a high schooler. Oh, my God."

Carol wanted to bolt. But she listened to the voice inside—one of her angels—who said, *You can do this. Just tell the truth and don't hold back, Gary needs you.*

The judge had Carol sworn in and said, This is on the record. This emergency hearing is being held for Gary Brian Stern to see if he is eligible for state assistance. Mr. Stern is being represented by Fred London's office and by Mrs. Stern. This is a formal hearing. The first thing I would like to do is hear from Mrs. Stern.

Carol had a box full of medical bills, which she put on the table.

Where is Mr. Stern? the judge asked.

"I am Mrs. Stern," Carol said. "I have power of attorney."

Is he able to talk? The judge asked.

"He can talk," Carol said, "but he's not going to make any sense, because for the last two days, he's been talking to the wall, and he's been talking to his dead mom."

The judge said to Carol, Mrs. Stern, please tell me why we are here.

Carol explained that Gary got sick in May. He went into Sinai Hospital and five days later was discharged, only to get worse at home. Carol told the court that Gary had been in hospitals for over four months straight, having surgery after surgery, procedures after procedures, infections after infections, seizures after seizures.

"I'm sorry," Carol said, "but I need to get graphic so you can understand the severity of my husband's condition."

Carol offered the judge the folder with material documenting what Gary had been going through.

"Please, open to the first page," Carol said. "What you see there is a picture of my husband before he got sick."

Carol added: "I'm sorry to have to show these."

There were fifteen pages of photos of Gary after he had gotten sick, pictures of Gary lying in bed, his internal organs visible.

"My husband can only have four ounces of water a day," Carol said. "He looks at his intestines moving around outside of his stomach and the pain— oh, the pain is so intense it's debilitating. This is a man who, before he got sick, showered twice a day; and now he needs me to wipe feces off of his stomach. He has a central line through which I feed him TPN every twelve hours."

The state attorney had tears in her eyes.

The judge also had tears in her eyes.

Carol's inner voice repeated, *Don't hold back.*

"Gary needs TPN because he can't digest food," Carol told the court. "If Gary drinks water, you will see it come out in his exposed internal organs forty-five seconds later."

Carol couldn't hold back her tears.

"My husband has to have more surgeries," Carol said. "He's going to be on TPN for a long time. It's expensive, and we have no insurance. We have no money. If I don't get help, my husband is going to die."

"I looked at the attorneys across from me," Carol said. "They were sniffling and wiping their eyes. The judge was blowing her nose."

The judge told Carol it normally took ninety days to get the response, but she promised it would not be that long.

"Her voice," Carol said, "was cracking."

Take care of yourself, the judge told Carol. It doesn't seem like I have to tell you to take care of your husband. From where I sit, you're already doing that.

They all walked out.

One state attorney told Carol off the record that that was by far the hardest hearing they'd been a part of. I hope the best for you and Mr. Stern.

# 43

Nine days later, Gary and Carol got a letter from the judge. Gary had won his state disability case, with Medicaid allowed to help pay the hospital bills and Equinox.

"The lawyers told me no one had ever gotten so quick a response before," Carol said.

Now, they had to fight in federal court to get social security disability, which would help cover all the other expenses. Carol said, "We were having a great day. We wanted to tell everybody, but who first?"

Carol's phone rang. It was David. Carol held out the phone and said, "You tell him."

"No," Gary said. "You tell him."

"Put it on speaker. We'll both tell. We're 50/50, remember."

They laughed.

"What's going on?" David asked.

"Carol did the impossible," Gary said. "I have Medicare."

"What's next?" David asked.

# 44

Kenny had been going back and forth from Baltimore to his home in North Carolina. In Baltimore, he took care of the dogs and worked on the four-story townhouse where Gary had lived for nineteen years.

Kenny had the top two floors cleaned, packed up, painted, and had moved Gary's hospital bed upstairs.

Carol bought voluminous night-gowns for Gary to wear (they are more comfortable and less likely to betray the bags beneath).

Gary was allowed four ounces of water a day. He was allowed two ices a day. He liked blueberry.

"He would be eating the blueberry ice," Carol said, "and all of a sudden, you would see Hermie, within thirty seconds, turn blue."

When Gary made a sarcastic joke, Carol figured it was a good sign.

Everyone was so happy about Gary being home, one of the neighbors made brownies, not realizing Gary couldn't eat. Gary watched Carol put the brownies—which Gary thought smelled as good as anything he had ever smelled—into the refrigerator. She stepped out the front door for five minutes for a smoke. When she came back inside, she went to drain Gary's Foley Bag.

"I saw what looked like coffee grounds," Carol said.

She asked Gary if he felt okay.

He said he was fine.

"It looks like you're bleeding internally," Carol said.

Then, she remembered the brownies.

"Did you eat the brownies?" she asked. "He told me noooo."

"If you didn't," Carol said, "you're bleeding. And if you're bleeding, I'm taking you to the hospital."

"I guess I can't get away with anything," Gary said.

"Nope," Carol said. "And you just used your Get Out Of Jail Free card."

Gary didn't say anything.

"I'm only doing this to keep you alive," Carol said. "You have to trust me."

"I trust you," Gary said. "I won't do it again."

It became a running joke. When he was finally able to eat, Carol got him a brownie with chocolate icing.

When Jade came to visit with Kenny, she was examining Gary's Foley Bag. She asked Pop Pop why the bag was turning blue. Carol shot a glance at Kenny, who said, "Let her see it."

Gary and Carol had been worried about Jade seeing Gary—her Pop Pop —in his condition, with his belly opened. But, if she found it disturbing, she didn't show it.

When she was introduced to Hermie, Jade said. "Yeah. Hermie the Crab."

Once, while Jade was helping Carol change the fistula bag, Jade said, "Hermie sure is crabby today."

Gary teased Jade with his pill trick. He swallowed a pill, which seconds later was visible inside his body, sitting on an internal organ.

Jade stayed for four days. While she was there, Gary was happy.

# 45

On December 23, 2011, Gary started throwing up and couldn't stop. Carol called the doctor and explained the situation.

At University Hospital, Dr. Chun asked how Gary was. As usual, Gary was in pain.

And he needed to get his gall bladder removed, which—Dr. Chun explained—couldn't be done until Gary's reconstruction.

The plastic surgeon, Dr. Holton, found out that Gary smoked, not very much, but occasionally.

Dr. Holton consequently put surgery off until the end of January—a good idea, Dr. Chun thought.

*More delay,* Carol thought.

# 46

On Christmas Day, Carol took Gary home for a few days so he could see the little tree she had decorated at the house.

"Everyone asked me how Gary's doing," Carol said. "They didn't really want to know. I would always say that he had good days and bad days. But truly he had good moments and bad moments. Mostly bad."

Carol made sure Gary got to his appointments with Dr. Chun and Doctor Cross—who were pleased with Gary's progress—although pain medication became an issue.

On one visit, Dr. Chun asked Gary how he was doing.

"I'm hurting," Gary said.

We'll get you some more pain medicine, Dr. Chun said. How else are you doing?

"I'm ready for surgery."

Not yet, Dr. Chun said. However, your abdomen is looking good. Dr. Chun looked at Carol and asked how she had managed to get Gary's abdomen to look so good.

Carol said, "A lot of TLC."

"She takes really good care of me," Gary said.

Dr. Chun sent Gary home to rest before his big surgery, which was scheduled for 8:00 in the morning, which meant they had to be there at 6:00. Carol got up at 4:30. She had a cup of coffee, a cigarette, got dressed, and took the dogs out for a walk.

About 5:15—it was still dark—she got Gary up and put him into the van.

"You all right?" she asked.

"You?" Gary asked back.

"I'm a little nervous," Carol said, "but I know everything's gonna be okay."

"I'm terrified," Gary said. "If something happens to me, I want you to—"

"You're going to be great," Carol said. "Nothing bad is going to happen to you." Then the lights in the van went out—both the inside lights and the headlights. She didn't know why. But it didn't seem like a good sign.

"Shit," Carol thought, driving blind. "Gary and I have been waiting so long for this day."

Carol got behind an eighteen-wheeler and used the truck to guide her. When she pulled up in front of the University of Maryland Hospital, the guy from valet parking went to get a wheelchair.

"I'm going to walk into this hospital," Gary said, "and I'm going to walk out."

Carol took Gary's walker from the back of the van. She disconnected Gary's IV lines, got him out of the van, put his Foley bags on the front of the walker, and covered him with his robe.

Taking small steps, bent over the walker, and shaky, Gary walked through the front doors of the hospital.

# 47

David and Stacey met Carol forty-five minutes before Gary went into surgery. They were all in pre-op together. Gary said he wanted to be alone with David for a few minutes. Carol gave Gary a kiss and said, "I'll see you when you get out. I love you."

Carol and Stacey went into the waiting room.

Carol remembers nothing about the next four and a half hours—until Dr. Chun came out.

Gary is doing great, Dr. Chun said. His ileostomy—the stoma, the opening in Gary's body—is gone and his gallbladder is out and his intestines are reconnected.

"So," David asked, "are you done?"

I'm done, Dr. Chun said. Dr. Holton is working on him now. Gary should be in there for a couple more hours.

Three hours later, Dr. Holton came out and announced that Gary was doing fine.

So, David said, it's all done, it's all over?

Well, no, Dr. Holton said. I had to put a Vac on Mr. Stern.

What? Carol asked.

Mr. Stern has a lot of scar tissue, Dr. Holton said. His abdomen has been through a lot so I have decided to give his body some more time. To heal.

My plan is to do a skin graft in a few days, maybe a week, Dr. Holton said.

They were going to be taking skin from other parts of Gary's body.

Ten days later, Dr. Holton told them Gary needed another week in the hospital.

"Gary was getting upset," Carol said. Very upset.

*Doesn't it ever end?*

"The doctors are not going to do a skin graft for at least another week," Carol told Kenny over the phone.

"Does Gary know?" Kenny asked.

"He's depressed about it," Carol said.

"He needs to see Jade," Kenny said.

Kenny arranged for Jade to be in Baltimore the next day.

Carol didn't tell Gary. After all the unhappy surprises, she wanted it to be a happy surprise. The next day, Kenny brought Jade, who put on a stethoscope and pretended to be a doctor.

Carol thought she would be better than many of the doctors who treated Gary.

## 48

After about a week, Dr. Holton did the skin graft, using skin from Gary's left leg. Gary felt as if his leg was on fire.

Dr. Holton did not close up Gary completely, but enough for him to go home. The plan was to let him heal where he'd be comfortable before coming back to the hospital for another plastic surgery to finish closing Gary's abdomen.

Gary no longer had a fistula bag or an ileostomy bag. No more Hermie. Even though Gary's skin graft was only a thin layer of skin, his intestines were back inside his stomach.

"Gary was moving around better," Carol said. "We could go anywhere."

But she was terrified, especially when Gary was standing up. What if Gary had a seizure and fell? If he did, would his stomach burst open? It would be a horror in any case, but if it happened in public Gary's humiliation would be insufferable.

Carol prayed that this time, Gary was home to stay, home to heal.

## 49

The first night at home, Carol was changing Gary's abdomen dressing. She was wiping his stomach when she saw green bubbles in Gary's wound. Another fistula, Carol knew. A bad sign. Carol didn't want to show her alarm, so she continued changing the dressing as if nothing was wrong.

Kenny had just reached North Carolina, when Carol contacted him, saying he had to turn around and come back to Baltimore: She needed him again. She also texted David, who said he would be there in five. Once David arrived to keep an eye on Gary, Carol went upstairs so Gary wouldn't overhear her call to Dr. Chun.

Carol told Dr. Chun that Gary had another fistula.

Dr. Chun asked if she was sure.

"Dr. Chun . . . " Carol started.

Yes, yes, Dr. Chun said. I know you're sure. Is he running a temperature?

"No," Carol said. "But you know Gary's body doesn't play by the rules."

<u>Do you think he should come back tonight?</u>

"No," Carol said. "Gary doesn't know."

<u>He needs to come back tomorrow morning,</u> Dr. Chun said.

When Kenny returned, David went home.

Gary wanted to know why Kenny was back. Kenny looked at Carol. He could tell by her look that Gary didn't know.

Carol was hiding a lot of bad news from Gary, to save him worry. She told him, "Kenny is coming back up to help me with the dogs, and to help me with the house."

"Did he bring Jade back?" Gary asked.

"Not this time," Carol said.

"Gary looked so sad," Carol said.

"Jade can't take time off from school," Carol explained.

Jade's school was all year round.

"Okay," Gary said. "Pack a bowl."

Carol nodded okay and told Kenny, "I need Gary to have one good night."

The next morning, Carol told Gary about the fistula and that he had to go back to the hospital. Gary started to cry, but in the middle of his sobbing he had a seizure.

Kenny called 911, which took Gary back to Sinai, where the doctors had been fixated on Crohn's. Only Dr. Antwi Kofi-Owusu—an internist who went to the University of the Caribbean School of Medicine—listened to Carol.

"He was one of the most compassionate doctors Gary ever had," Carol said.

Dr. Owusu became both Carol and Gary's primary care physician. He helped arrange Gary's move back to University of Maryland Hospital, where he was treated for the seizures.

Gary was put on the tenth floor on the other side of the hospital, an old part of University Hospital.

*The psych ward,* Carol figured. She was enraged.

"David," Gary told his brother, "these fucking people are making me crazy. I know I'm not an easy patient, but I'm going more crazy listening to the crazy people scream."

"The doctors and nurses on that floor are all the rejects," Carol said. "It was also the floor where the jail patients were kept. It was behind bars."

Gary wasn't the best patient.

Once Carol arrived to see a doctor running down the hall. Gary was behind him, yelling at him and throwing his IV pole at him.

"What's going on?" Carol asked Gary.

The doctor accused Gary of being in the hospital only to get pain medication.

"I'm not sure who was more pissed off," Carol said, "the doctor, Gary, or me."

Another time Carol walked into Gary's room and saw that Gary was connected to an IV pump, but there was no fluid in the line. It would have pumped air into Gary's heart.

"I cut that shit off right away," Carol said.

The next day, a code blue went off for the patient across the hall. The patient died. The code blue patient had Gary's nurse, the one who had almost pumped air into Gary's veins.

# 50

On Gary and Carol's anniversary, Dr. Chun told Gary he could go home, but that he still couldn't eat. Five weeks later, after Chun checked him out, he gave Gary the go-ahead to eat, but small bites only. No more than four ounces.

Carol went outside to have a smoke. When she went back into Gary's room, Gary was sitting up on the side of the bed, holding a dozen yellow roses. "You're not the only one who can do the impossible," Gary said. "Happy anniversary, Baby Doll."

*Gary just called me Baby Doll,* Carol thought. *He hasn't called me Baby Doll since before he got sick. OMG, it's our anniversary.*

It was close to Mother's Day. When they got home, Kimberly sent Carol some chocolate-covered strawberries.

"I don't have to tell you who got into them," Carol said.

"A strawberry is less than four ounces," Gary said.

"But," Carol said, "you ate twelve of them."

Gary was sick for the next two days.

Gary was going to the bathroom by himself, though he was supposed to wake Carol up when he did so, just in case. One night, Carol woke up with Butchy pulling the covers off her.

"I was sleeping on an air mattress," Carol said, "so I could be next to Gary."

Carol sat up. Confused by sleep and Butchy, who was acting, she realized, like Lassie. Butchy looked at Carol, then looked at the bathroom door. Once, twice, three times. He looked at Carol. He looked at the bathroom door. Then, the dog started to make crying sounds. Carol ran into the bathroom, where Gary was getting sick. Butchy stood next to Gary, looking at him with what Carol thought was a scared look.

Carol cleaned Gary up. She wiped his face with a cold wash cloth.

"Butchy," Gary said, "good boy. Good boy. I'm okay. I'm okay."

"Did you tell Butchy to get me?" Carol asked.

"No," Gary said. "I just started feeling like I was going to pass out."

"How are you now?" Carol asked.

"I'm just tired," Gary said.

"Let's get you back in bed," Carol said.

She stayed up the rest of the night watching Gary, but not alone. Butchy wouldn't take his eyes off him.

Five days later, Carol noticed Butchy staring at Gary, then looking over at her.

"What, Lassie?" Carol asked, "Has Timmy fallen down the well?"

Butchy started crying.

Gary looked down at Butchy and started to ask 'Butchy, what's . . .'

Before Gary could finish asking, his head went back, bubbles coming out of his mouth and nose, and his body went stiff. Carol tried to make sure Gary didn't hurt himself, to make sure he didn't choke. It took fifteen minutes for Gary to get back to normal. Carol was shaking.

"Butchy," Carol said, "Daddy's okay now."

The dog looked at her.

"Butchy," Gary said, "I'm okay."

Butchy started jumping and running around as if he knew he had just saved Gary's life.

# 51

Around the end of May 2012, Carol went out to get the mail, which included a letter from SSI. This time, Carol didn't wait to open it, fearing it was another denial letter. But Gary had won in state court, which meant that Social Security Income (SSI) would cover his hospital bills. But they needed help from the Federal Government to get Social Security Disability.

"I was really getting sick of this bull," Carol said. "I called my mom."

"It's time to get public opinion on our side," Jeanette said. "Have you called the Governor or the Congressman?"

"I spoke to the Governor," Carol said, "but not in the last couple of months."

"And the Congressman?"

"Not yet."

"Start with the Governor," Jeanette said, "and let him know you're going to call the Congressman."

Play them off against each other, see who wants to use helping Gary as good public relations—or who wants to avoid an accusation of inaction.

"I'm going to work on something," Jeanette said, "and I'll call you back."

Carol started calling politicians, starting with the mayor, Stephanie Rawlings-Blake, who told Carol, "There's nothing I can do. [W]e cannot declare him disabled."

Carol and David discussed having a GoFundMe account or an Indiegogo account, where people could donate money to help with Gary's care.

"I was willing to do anything at this point," Carol said.

Everyone in the family had a different idea of how to get public opinion on their side.

"It became a family fight." Carol said. "David, Stacey, Barbara, my mom, Linda, the Church, my kids, we even had people in the Netherlands, Germany, and Canada weighing in with their opinions.

Carol contacted *20/20*, *60 Minutes*, *Dr. Phil*, *Dr. Oz*, and *Fox News*.

"I even emailed *The View*" Carol said. "One of Gary's favorite shows."

No one responded.

"Let's go to YouTube," Kevin said. "We make a video. Pictures of you and Gary before and after he got sick. I can pull it together and put it to music. . . And shame the government into helping."

It took Kevin a week to produce the video; the before and after was heartbreaking, excruciating to watch. Kevin named the video: "His Life Is Worth Saving." Carol didn't like the title.

Carol and Kevin were on the phone, trying to figure out what more they could do. Gary was watching TV. The news came on, all about how President Obama was trying to get Obamacare passed and how Obama cared about his people.

"Let see how much Obama cares," Carol said.

They changed the title to "Obama Care? No, Obama Doesn't Care."

Carol asked Gary what he thought.

"It's good," Gary said, "but what is it going to do?"

"It's going to make our government stand up and take notice," Carol said. That's "when . . . [the politicians] started getting back in touch with me real fast," Carol said.

# 52

The White House got back to her.

"Is President Obama going to talk to me now?" Carol asked.

No, the White House representative said, I am.

It was, Carol thought, not that different from when she was a kid and answered the telephone call from Nixon. Except *this* time she wasn't joking.

The White House aide said, I'm here to tell you that you need change your YouTube video, or it's coming down.

"Go ahead and take it down," Carol said. "But I'm putting it right back up in bolder letters, and this time I'm going to contact the media. I'm an American citizen. I'm not going to say anything that's not true. But, if I have to, hell, I'll take it to the Supreme Court. I'm fighting for my husband's life."

<u>Are you going to change the post?</u> the White House representative demanded. <u>Or take it down?</u>

"You guys don't understand," Carol yelled. "You"—the government—"work for me. I don't work for you. You work for me and my husband. We put you in office, we'll take you out."

"I guess they weren't used to that," Carol later said. "I guess they were used to people, you know, getting bullied by them and cowering down, and that's not how I was taught. I was a military brat."

"Who's going to call me?" Carol asked the White House flack. "I need some answers."

Sometime later, two men appeared at Gary and Carol's front door.

"They didn't show ID," Carol said, "but they had black suits on. I knew where they were from. They weren't FBI. I've messed with the CIA before. My uncle was in the CIA for years."

"I'm not letting you in," Carol said. "This house is sanitized."

She had a sign on the front door: *Please, wash and sanitize hands, and put on a mask before entering this house.*

Carol figured they were crooked—everyone in the government on both sides of the aisle was crooked.

"The insurance companies run America," Carol said. "Obamacare was all about the insurance companies."

"Trumpcare"—what little Carol could figure out about it—"doesn't care either."

"I'm taking care of my husband," Carol told the two men. "Nothing is going to change, and there's nothing you can do about it."

Carol told them, "When I start getting phone calls from people telling me things are going to change, then I'm going to change my attitude."

"The next day, I got another phone call from the White House," she said, and that was promising.

Nothing definite, but it was a response.

She also got a letter, which said she would be getting a phone call from some senators and Congressmen who—Carol said—claimed they were taking care of Gary's situation. State Senator Eileen Brooke gave me a name of an attorney and rushed us to the courthouse."

Stacey came over to watch Gary, while Carol went out to do battle with the government.

"I needed to make sure that Gary's medication was paid for," Carol said. "I couldn't expect the church in Martinsburg, West Virginia, to keep paying for it. It's not like those people had a lot of money, and they were giving and giving to me all the time. I needed to try and take care of it myself."

Once the government started helping, Carol called [her brother] and said, "Change the post from 'Obama Doesn't Care' to 'Please Save My Pop-Pop's Life.' And she wanted him to put up a warning: "Extremely Graphic."

She continued to get government responses, "making sure that everything was okay," Carol said, "because they knew I was serious, and I wasn't going to stop."

And, if Carol ever thought about stopping, her angels wouldn't let her.

# 53

"Mom always changed her pictures around," Carol said.

One time, when Gary and Carol visited Jeanette in West Virginia, Carol hugged Willem and started down the hall to Jeanette's bedroom.

"Gary and Pop stayed in the living room," Carol said. "I wasn't thinking about much of anything, but was just happy to be there."

At the end of the hall was a picture Carol had never seen before, or didn't recall ever seeing.

"The woman in the picture was my angel," Carol said.

Carol stood still, transfixed, recalling the first time her angel had visited her.

"Her hair, her dress . . . " Carol said. "I have no idea how long I stood there."

Jeanette called from her bedroom.

"I walked into her bedroom," Carol said. "I didn't even hug her before I asked, "Mom where did you get the picture from?"

"What picture?" Jeanette asked.

"The one hanging in the hall."

"You mean the one of my mother. Your Aunt Gwen sent it to me a few weeks ago. Beautiful, isn't it?"

"Yes, she was. Have I ever seen it before?"

"No, honey. Your Uncle Garald had it. When he passed away, your Aunt Gwen got it and sent it to me."

"So I've never seen it before?"

"I don't see how you could've. You've never been to your Uncle Garald's place."

"Mom, that's a picture of my angel. The one that came to me after dad was missing."

"Are you sure?"

"That's her," Carol said.

"I always knew she stayed close to us," Jeanette said.

# 54

During the summer and fall of 2012, because Gary was home, it was increasingly hard to protect him from finding out how broke they were. Every day brought more bills.

And Gary was getting sicker. Over the next nine months he was in hospitals over a dozen times for various procedures, for seven weeks at University Hospital, for more reconstruction. Many of the surgeries involved more resection of both his large and small bowel; he didn't have a lot of bowel left.

*Never let Gary see her feel any disgust with anything having to do with Gary.*

Carol faced facts. Gary's medical odyssey was not necessarily going to have a happy ending.

"I'm getting tired of this shit," Gary said.

"What's new?" David asked.

"It's funny you should ask that," Carol said, "because the nurses at Northwest took me aside and said I should look into Gary's medical record."

"I've been telling you they screwed up," Gary said.

"We knew that when you were in Northwest the first time," David said.

David and Stacey took turns coming over and giving Carol a break so she could shower and try to sleep, although she was having trouble sleeping and sometimes didn't get any rest for days. Mostly, when David and Stacey helped, Carol went out to shop for food or medical supplies.

And Gary's pain was getting worse, off the one-to-ten chart.

# 55

---

Gary was on the tenth floor. Dr. Chun planned to take him to the OR on Monday for a washout. Carol was outside smoking when she got a call from Gary, who said, "I need you up here now. This damned doctor"—not Dr. Chun—"came in my room, and he said I can't get any more liquid IV pain medication. He said he was discharging me so I needed to start on pills."

"The doctor has you confused with another patient," Carol said.

"He knows who I am," Gary said.

"Then," Carol said, "he's got to know you're going to the OR on Monday for a washout."

"He said Dr. Chun changed his mind."

Carol hurried to Gary's room and asked him, "Where is this doctor."

"He's a redhead," Gary said.

Carol found the doctor, a third-year intern, in the nurses' station.

"Excuse me," Carol said, "are you the one who just came out of my husband's room?"

Who is your husband? the redhead asked.

"Mr. Stern."

Yes, I was.

"I would like to talk to you."

Go ahead.

"Somewhere more private."

Your husband's room.

"How about this corner?" Carol indicated a spot where they weren't likely to be disturbed. Carol is five feet tall. The redhead was over six feet. Standing toe-to-toe, Carol looked up into the redhead's face.

"Did you tell my husband he was going on pill medication?" Carol asked.

<u>Yes,</u> the redhead said. <u>I did.</u>

"Why did you tell him that?"

"He's been on IV medicine too long, and we are discharging him tomorrow."

"First of all, it is not up to you to take my husband off IV meds. Second of all, until I hear from Dr. Chun, my husband is not going anywhere ."

<u>Anything else?</u>

"Yes, you upset my husband, therefore you have lost the right to speak to him."

Carol went back into Gary's room. It took her two hours to calm him down. When he finally drifted off, Carol went out to have a smoke. She wasn't downstairs for more than ten minutes when Gary again called her.

"Carol," Gary said, "he"—the redhead—"was just back in here and told me he didn't care what you said, he's going to change the orders on my meds."

When Carol told Gary she'd take care of it immediately, Gary said, "It won't do any good. He told me he was leaving the floor."

"Don't you worry," Carol said. "I know where he's going."

Carol went inside to the security guards, whom she had gotten to know.

"You're probably going to get a call about a hysterical woman on WB5," she told the security guards. "It's going to be me. Do me a favor, I know you have to come up, but please give me ten minutes before you do."

<u>What's going on?</u> one of the security guards asked.

"No one messes with Gary," Carol said. "I'm going to have some intern's ass."

<u>Go get him,</u> the security guard said.

Carol figured the redhead was going to be in the office on WB5, but she found him still in the nurses' station, where she confronted him.

"We need to go somewhere and talk," Carol told him.

<u>We can talk right here,</u> the redhead said.

"If you don't care, I don't care."

The redhead just sat there.

"I told you that you were not allowed to speak to my husband."

<u>You're not my patient. Your husband is.</u>

"Pick up the phone and call Dr. Chun."

<u>I can't.</u>

"What do you mean you can't?"

<u>I can't.</u>

"You can pick up that phone and call Dr. Chun or—

From her back pocket, Carol took out her phone and showed it to him.

"I guarantee if Dr. Chun sees my number, he *will* pick it up."

He's in the OR.

"He takes his phone with him to the OR, and he will answer it."

The redhead picked up the nurses' station phone and started calling.

"Put it on speaker," Carol said.

Dr. Chun answered. On speaker.

"Dr. Chun," Carol said.

Hello, Carol, what's up?

"Can you please explain to your third-year intern who is in charge of my husband's care."

The only one who makes decisions or speaks to Mr. Stern is Mrs. Stern or myself.

After the phone call was over, Carol said to the redhead, "Do you understand you have not only lost the privilege of speaking to my husband, you have also lost the privilege of going into his room."

Behind the redhead, half the staff were laughing.

"And that," Carol said, "was the last time I had a problem with a doctor in that hospital."

# 56

"What happened next is hard to think about," Carol said, "but it's time . . . "

Dr. Chun did exploratory surgery, put a Vac back on Gary, and ordered regular washouts.

Gary's white count climbed higher and higher. They kept putting Jackson-Pratt (JP) tubes into him to see what was going on inside his body cavity.

Gary had five JP (Jackson-Pratt) drains snaking from his body. He also had an IR drain, which is almost the same as JP drain but with bigger tubes.

Gary looked like an octopus.

"David did the same thing I did," Carol said. "We didn't let anyone else disturb Gary with their reactions. David threw people out of the room if they would start to say the wrong thing, start to react the wrong way, or if they would come in with food and water. And it didn't matter who it was. They would have to leave."

Gary's Vac was leaking, irritating Gary's skin. Gary's temperature was low, but his white cell count was high, which didn't make sense. A high white cell count meant Gary had an infection, which presumably would send his temperature up. His heart rate was high, but his blood pressure was low. Another conundrum.

On February 20, 2013, Gary didn't get out of post-op until after midnight. He had gotten about three, maybe four hours of sleep, and then he woke up screaming.

The anesthesiologist ordered more pain medication to make Gary comfortable. Gary calmed down—briefly, before the pain hit him again. The next day, Gary started running a fever.

Dr. Chun and Dr. Cross told Carol they had started Gary on antibiotics to help Gary kick the infections that were causing pain. They sent Gary down for more testing.

Always more tests.

Dr. Cross told Carol they needed to put contrast in Gary's NG tube (the one that went through the nose into the stomach).

After the doctors left, Carol went back into the room. Watching Gary suffer, Carol despaired.

*When would this horror end?*

Gary was pretty out of it, but Carol was sure he understood what she was saying.

"They're going to take you down for some test," Carol said. "I'm going to run home and check on the dogs. "

Gary managed to murmur, "Okay, love."

Carol was walking to the elevator—it was a long hallway—when she heard one of her angels telling her, *Don't go.*

Carol kept walking.

*Don't go,* the voice repeated.

Carol slowed down, but kept heading to the elevators until she felt a hand on her left shoulder.

Carol spun around.

No one was there.

When Carol turned back toward the elevators, she felt two hands on her back, which pushed her.

Again, Carol turned around.

Again, no one was there.

Carol went back to Gary's room, which was the last room on the left side of the floor. Gary's eyes were closed. Carol thought he was sleeping. Someone put hands on her cheeks and moved her head down toward Gary's stomach.

"I started looking at his JP tube when a nurse's assistant came in," Carol said. "I tried to look up at her, but my head wouldn't move."

The fluid coming through Gary's tube turned green.

"I couldn't believe what I was looking at," Carol said.

Carol thanked God that Gary was asleep.

At the nurses station, Carol said, "I need Gary's doctor. "

The doctors will be up after Mr. Stern's test results come in, the nurse said.

"I need them now," Carol said.

They can't come up right now, the nurse said.

Carol started pounding her fist on the nurse's station.

"I need the doctors now," Carol said, when Dr. Holton appeared, "walking up to me really fast."

He put his hand on Carol's arm above her elbow and walked her down the hallway.

"I need you to go into Gary's room," Carol said, "and look at the JP tube on the right side. Pick it up, pour it out, and smell it. If you can tell me that what we are looking at is all right, then you can do whatever test you want."

That sounds fair.

"One more thing," Carol said. "You can't let Gary know what you're looking at. I don't want him upset."

Dr. Holton agreed. He and the nurse followed Carol to Gary's room. He was awake. Dr. Holton walked up to the right side of Gary's bed. The nurse went up to the left. Carol stood at the foot of the bed.

Hi, Mr. Stern, Dr. Holton said. I'm just stopping by to see if you're feeling any better.

As he talked, he checked out Gary's JP tube. The nurse got a cup from the bathroom, which she handed to Dr. Holton.

As Dr. Holton made small talk to distract Gary, he poured some of the fluid from Gary's tube into the cup and sniffed it.

OR STAT, Doctor Holton told the nurse.

Gary was terrified. He had no idea what was going on. In a matter of minutes he had eight people in his room, everyone doing something different to him. Checking his vitals, giving him medicine through an IV, and getting him ready for new x-rays.

Gary was crying out Carol's name over and over. But she was outside the ring of doctors and nurses surrounding Gary, whom they soon wheeled away. Again.

Carol contacted David, who rushed to the hospital.

Four hours later, Dr. Chun and Dr. Holton came out of the OR together. Dr. Chun was shaking his head. Dr. Holton said if Carol had delayed even fifteen minutes or if Carol hadn't protested about putting contrast into Gary's NG, he would have died.

"You can think of the angels any way you want," Carol said. "Maybe woman's intuition, but I know in my heart and soul that the angels were just telling me what the next step was."

## 57

Dr. Chun believed it was time to try another skin graft. Carol and David weren't sure that was a good idea. Gary was feeling hopeless because of all the operations.

Gary's body kept rejecting skin grafts.

Let me look at your legs, Dr. Holton said to Gary. Was there skin he could use for the graft?

Dr. Holton's assistant checked Gary's legs.

I see a part right here where we can do another graft, the assistant said.

"I'll be damned if you're going to skin me alive," Gary said.

Carol started clapping.

"Good for you, Babe," she said. "I couldn't have said it better myself." To the assistant, Carol said, "Doctor, I suggest you find another way to put skin on my husband's body."

"Okay," he said, "we'll use a cadaver."

"Not a problem," Carol said.

The cadaver skin didn't work. They tried another cadaver, which also didn't work.

Carol was watching Gary go through so much pain, getting more and more depressed, but what could she do? She did what she always did, she prayed and then went outside for a smoke.

Carol and a second-year intern, Mike, had bonded over both being smokers.

"I'm really tired of Gary going into the OR's for washouts," Carol told him. "I think it's time we start doing bedside washouts."

She could do the washouts herself.

Carol explained to the intern what the problem was and her solution.

Surgical donuts—pads—cushioned the Vac but also irritated the skin.

"We're going to cut these donuts in half," Carol said. "We're going to measure them and put them around the fistulas."

Since Mike wanted to become a plastic surgeon and work with his dad in Massachusetts, he was open to trying Carol's method, which worked.

Gary started to come around. He liked Mike.

Carol would go into Gary's room and hear both Gary and Mike laughing. It was a good sound for Carol to hear.

One of the nurses came up to Carol and told her, Gary is worried about you, he thinks you're not eating. Are you eating?

"Sure, I am," Carol said. "How can I take food into Gary's room? To let him smell it, to watch me eat, its been so long since Gary had anything to eat."

Well, the nurse said, Gary has arranged for you to have a tray brought to his room three times a day for you to eat.

"Gary is lying in that bed not knowing if his going to live or die," Carol said, "and he's worried about me."

# 58

It seemed as if everything was under control—until March 18, 2013. About 9:30 a.m.

"Carol," Gary cried out, "my back, my back . . ."

Carol heard one of her voices saying, *Get the nurse now.*

Gary was gasping for breath.

Carol pushed the emergency button and told Gary, "Babe, I will be right back."

Carol ran down the hall. Five rooms down she found Gary's nurse.

"I need you in Gary's room," Carol said. "Gary can't breathe."

The nurse walked toward Gary's room. Slowly. At the door, he stopped to put on an isolation gown. Carol grabbed the gown and said, "Fuck the gown. Get in there. Now."

"This nurse had two speeds," Carol said. "Slow and slower."

Carol saw a blood pressure machine. And Denise, an LPN (licensed practical nurse) she trusted. Carol grabbed both and rushed both into Gary's room.

"Gary's not breathing right," Carol said. "Something's wrong."

He's tachycardic, Denise said. His respiration is shallow. Start oxygen.

Gary wasn't moving. Denise got on her phone and started talking to someone. Carol still thought that the response to Gary's condition wasn't fast enough, so she ran to a doctors' meeting room. She pounded on the glass door until one of the female doctors came out and asked Carol, "What's going on?"

"My husband," Carol couldn't get the words out. "My . . ."

Denise had walked up behind her and said to the doctor, I need you in twenty-seven, Gary's room, STAT. Immediately.

Denise and the doctor ran into Gary's room.

We need to call it, the doctor said.

*Call it?* Carol thought she was saying Gary was dead. But call it referred to Code Blue.

Everything Gary had gone through went through her head. All the surgeries, fistulas, TPN, seizures, bleeding out, intestines, blood clots, pain. . .

Her voice told her, *He will make it. Just pray.* Which is what Carol did.

Twenty people gathered in front of Carol. One of them asked Carol, Can I call anyone for you?

Carol gave the woman her cell phone and told her to call David.

*Code Blue WB5, Code Blue WB5* was still blaring out of the loud speakers.

More people—doctors, nurses, Carol didn't know who—were running into Gary's room with machines. Denise came out.

"Get Dr. Chun," Carol said. "I want Dr. Chun"—who at that moment came running up.

"I need you in there," Carol said.

That's respiratory, Dr. Chun said. I'd be in the way.

"They may be experts in their field," Carol said, "but you and I are the only experts on Gary. Just stand back so if they have any questions you can answer them."

Dr. Chun agreed and went into the room.

David hurried down the hall to Carol as the doctors and nurses wheeled Gary out, taking him to Shock Trauma ICU. Dr. Chun stayed with Gary, for hours.

The doctors and nurses had been worried that Gary might have gotten MRSA (Methicillin-resistant Staphylococcus aureus), an infection that spreads in hospitals.

When Dr. Chun came into the waiting room, he looked defeated.

Gary's okay, but it's a mess, Dr. Chun said.

He had four fistulas.

He has a Vac on, Dr. Chun said. I need to put him back in SICU (Surgical Intensive Care Unit). He's going to need washouts three or four times a week.

## 59

Anytime Gary was in SICU, ICU, or STICU, Carol couldn't stay with him. Carol would move everything she had in the room to her van, where she slept. Going home was not an option. She needed to stay close. *How is his white count? His potassium? What's his magnesium? His triglycerides? Is he getting a bedsore? Did he need another Vac change? How is his sugar? Did he get his pain medication? Did he get his seizure medication? How is his hemoglobin?*

"Why am I thinking and worrying about these things?" Carol wondered. Gary had doctors, nurses, and dietitians. Why did *she* have to stay on top of it all?

"They all had lots of patients," Carol said. "I had only one Gary, and I wasn't going to let them miss anything."

It had been three days since Gary had a Vac change. Carol was walking from the hospital elevator to the ICU when Dr. Chun called, asking where she was.

"I'm on my way to see Gary," Carol said. "Is he ok?"

It's time to do a Vac change, Dr. Chun said.

"I was just thinking about that," Carol said.

One of my interns is on her way to Gary's room to help you.

SICU have their own doctors and nurses and their own rules. Each SICU nurse cared for only two patients. Carol hurried to Gary's room, which was ten rooms down the hallway. Carol had just enough time to say good morning to Gary, who was awake.

"Where have you been?" Gary asked.

"You know I can't sleep in here," Carol said.

"Where have you been sleeping?"

"They have a family room with couches that open into beds. I've been sleeping there," Carol lied. She didn't want Gary to worry.

Five minutes later, David arrived and walked up to Gary's bed.

"Do you know where Carol has been sleeping?" Gary asked him.

"Oh, my God," Carol thought. "Don't tell him."

"Probably the waiting room."

*I dodged a bullet,* Carol thought.

Gary's nurse walked in. A new face. Carol introduced herself and David. The nurse didn't say much. He got Gary's vitals and left, passing one of Dr. Chun's interns.

"Are you ready to do this?" the intern asked.

Gary's washout.

"I don't have any supplies," Carol said. "I'm not used to this floor. I could go up to WB5 and get the supplies from up there."

The intern's phone rang. For privacy, the intern went behind the nurse's station.

The nurse who had taken Gary's vitals came back and asked Carol, What is this about?

"Vac change and washout," Carol said.

The nurse looked puzzled. He turned to walk away, but, after three steps, he turned back and walked up to Carol. Too close.

You're going to have to leave, he said.

"What?" Carol asked.

This is SICU, he said. We do not allow family members in the room when we do wash out.

Who's going to do it? Carol asked.

We will, the nurse said. You're going to have to—

Dr. Chun's intern had finished her phone call and asked the nurse, What are you doing?

I'm letting her know she has to leave until we get done, the nurse said. We can't let her assist in washouts.

What are you talking about, the intern asked. She's not assisting me. I'm assisting her.

I have to talk to my resident, the nurse said.

"Go ahead," Carol said.

The nurse walked over to a resident, who was sitting in front of a computer at the 2 nurses' station.

"I heard Gary's nurse say 'Mrs. Stern is here,'" Carol said.

The resident stood up real fast and asked, Where is she?

The nurse pointed at Carol.

Carol waved at him.

The resident walked toward her.

Mrs. Stern, the resident said. I spoke to Dr. Chun. I've been expecting you. It's a pleasure to meet you. You're notorious at this hospital. The things you've accomplished. Anything you need, anything, just ask.

"As a matter fact," Carol said, "I need supplies for a washout and Vac change. And I need to make sure Gary has plenty of pain medication."

No problem, the resident said. Anything else?

"Well, yes." Carol pointed at the nurse. "Will you let him know it's okay for me to be in here and do this."

You give her anything she asks for, the resident told the nurse. No questions asked.

To Carol, the resident said, <u>Mrs. Stern, do you mind if some of my</u> <u>interns come to the room so they can learn from you how to do a proper</u> <u>wash out and Vac change?</u>

"Sure," Carol said. "It's going to take me an hour to set up before I start."

David, who was listening from inside Gary's room, laughed.

Carol's procedure ended up being used by others.

# 60

Putting suction on the fistulas helped keep Gary's insides clean, but the suction of the Vac made more holes.

"A Catch-22," Carol said.

Part of Gary's abdomen needed suction and part of it couldn't have suction. But the new kind of donut Carol had designed was helping.

"How many of my interns can watch you," a resident asked.

"I don't care," Carol said. "I can explain what I'm doing and why I'm doing it if you would like."

"When would you like them in here?" The resident asked.

"Well, the prep is just as important if not more so," Carol said. "If you'd like them in now, have them come in."

A half dozen interns gathered around as she and David worked. They asked questions such as "Why use silverdine [a white antimicrobial cream]?" "How many fistulas does he have?" And "Where do you practice medicine?"

A doctor told Carol, "You know what, I never let family members in. But you, I'd like in every room with me, and if I ever need an advocate, I want permission to call you."

"Sorry," Carol said, "but I only take care of my best friend. My love. My Gary."

That's how Carol left it.

"It was nice that he was good with the fact that I was making it more comfortable for my husband, which was the only thing I wanted to do," Carol said.

It wasn't yet about becoming a patient advocate. It wasn't about the doctors. It wasn't about Carol.

"It was," Carol said, "all about Gary."

Patients who don't have someone like Carol when they're in the hospital —no close friends or family to argue for them—don't necessarily make it.

"They may make it a couple months," Carol said, "but they can be ignored, uncomfortable, abandoned."

Gary was moved back to WB5.

# 61

Two of Dr. Chun's interns came in to help Carol with a Vac change and washout. Gary was more heavily sedated than usual.

"David and Stacey were there," Carol said, "so I'm pretty sure it was a Saturday."

When the second intern pulled off the foam protecting Gary's organs, Carol said, "Oh, my God." Her body went ice cold.

"If at any time I was going to pass out, this was the time," Carol said. "I'm sure I wasn't the only one."

Carol looked from the mess that was Gary's stomach to David, who saw fear in Carol's eyes. He edged up to the bed and looked at Gary's stomach. Carol could see fear in his eyes.

Dr. Chun entered the room and took one look at Carol's face, and then looked down at Gary's stomach.

"That day," Carol said, "Dr. Chun couldn't manage a poker face."

Carol counted fourteen fistulas. When the Vac had been attached, there had been only four—"which meant," Carol said, "there were fourteen big areas of Gary's small intestines that had gastric content coming out.

Dr. Chun told his interns not to put the Vac back on but to put a fistula bag on instead.

He then looked at Carol as if to say *let's go into the hallway*, which they did.

Dr. Chun asked, "Carol, are you all right?"

"Dr. Chun," Carol said, "I'm the most selfish person in the world. Gary wanted to die, and I told him to keep fighting."

Dr. Chun put his hands on her shoulders.

Listen to me, Dr. Chun said. Gary is alive because of you. He may say he wants to die, but he doesn't. He wants to fight for you. He wants to live for . . . both of you.

"Is he going to die?" Carol asked.

He's not going to live to be 94, Dr. Chun said. But we will get him through this, you and me. We will do this.

"We can do this?" Carol asked.

Gary loves you, Dr. Chun said. Nothing is going to stop him.

The next few days Carol and David did everything they could to make sure Gary did not see how bad his stomach was. Whenever Gary started to look down at himself, Carol or David would distract him by talking or making noise. When it was time to change his fistula bag, they put up a sheet blocking his view. Carol would station a nurse next to the head of the bed and engage him in a conversation. This went on for five days.

"I don't know how much longer we can keep this from him," Carol told David.

"You think we should tell him?" David asked.

"I don't know," Carol said. "I don't know how he's going to handle it."

"It's better we tell him first," David said.

"You're right," Carol said. "But how do you tell Gary after everything he's gone through?"

"I'll get him high," David said. "Then, you tell him."

When they went back into Gary's room, Gary was awake.

"Hey, Babe," Carol said, "David is going to stay in here for five minutes. I will be in the hallway."

"Sounds good," Gary said, suspecting David had brought him marijuana for the pain.

Carol didn't do drugs, but to make Gary easy, she pretended to smoke.

"It was just a bad situation," Carol said.

"I was standing in the hallway thinking about how I was going to tell Gary, how I was going to put it," Carol said. "Do I just come out with it? Do I ease into it?"

She forgot she was keeping watch. When Dr. Chun walked up, she started to open the door for him. Inside Gary was coughing.

"Oh, shit," Carol thought. "The weed."

She stopped short. Dr. Chun walked into her as she turned around.

"Dr. Chun," Carol said, "can we talk before we go in?"

"I don't remember what we talked about," Carol said. "It was about Gary, but I was just trying to stall. Maybe Dr. Chun was, too."

After a moment, they went in. The air reeked of marijuana. Dr. Chun didn't say anything. He asked how Gary was feeling.

"I'm all right," Gary said, "now."

"Good," Dr. Chun said, "we are coming up with a plan. You just rest." Dr. Chun left.

Gary and David were laughing.

Carol laughed, too. But she knew now was the time to tell Gary the bad news.

"You can't hide things from me as well as you think you can," Gary said. "Why didn't you say anything to me?"

"I didn't want to upset you," Carol said.

"We'll get through this," Gary said.

50/50.

Just like they had gotten through everything.

# 62

Carol caught up with Dr. Chun in the hall.

I'm thinking about letting you take Gary home, Dr. Chun said.

A few hours later, one of the GI doctors checked on Gary.

"Dr. Chun mentioned about taking Gary home," Carol said.

We've all discussed it, the GI doctor said.

"Is he going to be able to eat?" David asked.

Chances are he will never eat again, the GI doctor said.

"Why can't you do a transplant?" David asked.

We don't do transplants on intestines, the GI doctor said.

"You do it on everything else," David said.

Once again Carol's thought rushed. *Gary is in pain. Gary will never eat again. Gary's intestines are all outside his body. Gary is depressed. Gary is getting 12 mg. IV Dilaudid an hour. How can I keep him comfortable? What's going on with his labs? How do I keep him comfortable? How do I keep him happy? How do I stop him from eating?*

"I can do this," Carol said, "but how?"

# 63

---

"I need a cigarette," Carol told David. "I need to think."

David told her to go ahead. He'd hold down the fort.

Downstairs, Carol went out the side door and, skipping the hospital smoking area, crossed the street. She didn't want to run into anyone she knew.

"How," she wondered. . . "How do I do this."

The first thing she decided was that she needed to pray.

"Dear Heavenly Father," she prayed, "I know in my heart You have not left my side, and You have not left Gary's side. Well, I need you bad. I truly believe Gary would not be going through all this for no reason. I know you have a plan, and I know You have sent Your Angels to me. I'm not out here to ask why. I will not question You. I will ask for Your help. The doctors think I can get Gary better at home. But I don't know how. Please help me figure out how to do it. In the name of our Father and the son, and the Holy Ghost. Amen.

"Okay," Carol said to herself, "now I can think."

The biggest problem was Gary's pain medication.

"Just then." Carol said, "Jess, one of the OR LPNs, walked by."

She had hoped to avoid seeing anyone she knew, but was grateful for Jess's company.

Mrs. Stern, Jess asked. How is Mr. Stern?

Carol lost it. Jess sat down next to her and waited until she calmed down. She explained the situation.

Have you talked to the case manager? Jess asked.

Carol went inside. At the elevator were two women in suits with white scrubs over them. Carol didn't recognize them. At the fifth floor, Carol got off the elevator. They got off behind her. As Carol walked to WB5, she heard one of them say, It was a type of hospice . . .

Hospice? Carol thought.

She turned around and asked the two a dozen questions. They seemed to be experts in hospice care. One of them handed Carol her business card, took down Gary's information, and said she would look into his case.

"Serendipity?" Carol wondered. "Or arranged by one of my angels?"

Carol spoke to pain management, who said the only way to keep Gary on IV meds was in a hospice."

She spoke to David, to her mom, to one of her sisters, to her kids. She asked everyone what she should do.

Everyone said the same thing: she would make the right decision.

Carol asked everyone except the one that mattered the most—Gary.

"How do I ask him?" Carol said. "I'm not giving up, but, if I ask him, he will give up, because he will think I'm giving up."

For two days, Carol couldn't decide what to do.

"After months, and months, and months, this is it?" Carol thought. "This is how it ends?"

On the third day, Carol didn't even have a chance to put down her purse when Gary said, "I know what's going on."

"Babe," Carol said, "what are you talking about?"

"They want you to take me home."

Carol believed they could read each other's thoughts.

"We've been talking about it."

"How, why, when?"

"Dr. Chun feels I can take better care of you than they can."

"I could of told them that."

"We only have one problem."

"Pain medicine."

"I'm working on something now."

"You're thinking about hospice."

"I'm not taking you home to die."

Carol signed the papers to release Gary from the hospital.

"The Death Papers," Carol thought.

Carol signed and told Gary, "Let's go home."

# 64

Two days later, while Carol was talking to the hospice doctor, Dr. Chun came up and said, "Carol, hospice? Really?"

"Dr. Chun, look at Gary," Carol said. "Do you really think I can fix this at home without the proper pain medication? I'm telling you I can't. I'm telling you I want to, but if I'm not allowed to give him IV medication, I can't do it, and they're saying that I can't do it unless he's on hospice."

Gary was too young to be at hospice, Dr. Chun said. I'm not giving up.

Sending Gary to a hospice felt like giving up, an admission that Gary was going to die.

He told Carol he was going to track down a doctor who could do intestinal transplants. He had been in Pennsylvania, but was no longer in the area. Dr. Chun discussed Gary with Dr. Raymond Cross, a gerontologist, who was going to talk to a colleague in Pittsburgh who knew a doctor at the Cleveland Clinic—Dr. Kareem Abu-Elmagd. Everyone called him Dr. Kareem. He was a hepato-pancreato-biliary and transplant surgeon who might be able to transplant Gary's intestines and liver.

Dr. Chun spent the entire night and half the morning sending Gary's records to the Cleveland Clinic.

Dr. Kareem agreed to accept Gary, Dr. Chun said

Dr. Chun called Carol and asked where she was. She was right outside Gary's hospital room.

I'm four minutes away, Dr. Chun said, Stay there, I've got some news.

As usual, they met in the hallway outside of Gary's room—Carol's office—where Dr. Chun told Carol that Dr. Kareem had agreed to take on Gary.

Carol said, "Okay?" It was more a question than an agreement.

This means a lot of retesting for Gary, Dr. Chun said. A lot of work.

"This isn't my decision," Carol said. "It's Gary's."

Dr. Chun tore up the release papers she had signed.

Carol and Doctor Chun entered Gary's room together.

Gary—and David, who was with Gary—could tell something was up.

David went to one side of the bed while Carol and Dr. Chun stood at the foot of the bed.

Gary suspiciously eyed Dr. Chun. But when he glanced at Carol, who seemed calm, Gary figured whatever Dr. Chun was going to suggest would be okay.

Dr. Chun held Gary's hand and said, "Gary, we have an option here, but this option has got to come from only you. This isn't an option for you and Carol, this is an option for you."

Only Gary could decide.

"I don't understand," Gary said. "What are you talking about?"

We have made arrangements, Dr. Chun said. You can go on home, on hospice, and we can get you comfortable, but you're going to die.

Because Gary had been on TPN so long that some of his organs were starting to fail.

Or, Dr. Chun said, you can go to the Cleveland Clinic, where Dr. Kareem is [and] have an intestinal transplant . . . But they're going to have to do all these tests that you've gone through, that you hate so much, over again . . . [B]ut it's a chance for you to live and [for] you and Carol to have a normal life.

"Where are you going to be?" Gary asked Carol.

"Where on earth do you think I would be?" she said. "I'm going to be right by your side, every step of the way, I don't care where it is, I don't care if it's here, Cleveland, or across the world, I'm not leaving your side."

Gary said, "Let's go to Cleveland."

# 65

How could they get Gary from Baltimore to Cleveland?

"It's not like he can go down to BWI and jump on a plane," Carol said.

Carol couldn't sleep: *Where could she get the money to take Gary to Cleveland?*

Sunny, Gary's favorite nurse, woke Carol up at 5:30 that morning with a pot of coffee, a copy of Gary's latest labs, and a smile.

Gary just fell asleep, Sunny said.

After showering and dressing, Carol went to WB5 and had the charge nurse make a copy of Gary's labs.

After Carol had been attacked, she hadn't renewed her driver's license. Gary took her wherever she had to go, or she drove without a current license. But Carol needed a license so she had ID for the flight with Gary, and to change her name to Stern on her social security card.

The social security office was only five minutes from Carol's house, and Carol needed to make sure she was there with her marriage license when it opened at nine o'clock. By ten o'clock, as Carol was on her way to get her new driver's license, she got a call from the Cleveland Hospital, Dr. Kareem's office manager.

"I was expecting your call," Carol told the office manager.

We have a problem, the office manager said. Mr. Stern does not have Medicaid. He only has Medicare, and Medicare only works in the state you live in.

"Wait, no," Carol said. "That's not right. The Federal judge declared Gary disabled two weeks ago."

It takes sixty days before Medicaid takes effect, the office manager said. You have forty-five days to go.

"Gary doesn't have forty-five days," Carol said. "Please keep working on the paperwork. I promise I will call you back after I straighten out everything. Expect us in three days."

Carol pulled the van to the side of the road as once more her thoughts raced. *I can't believe this. Everything Gary has gone through, and now he can't go to Cleveland because it's forty-five days too early. It'll be forty-five days too late. I'm not going to let this happen.*

"When I called the Governor's office," Carol said, they told her, *call her Congressman . . . no, call her Senator.* "I called both of them 'the Congressman' and 'the senator.'"

The senator told her she had to talk to the Congressman. It wasn't a *state* issue.

The Congressman's assistant told Carol that the Congressman was in a meeting.

"This is Mrs. Stern," Carol said. "This is Gary Stern's wife, Carol Stern, I want to talk to him, and I want to talk to him now. I'm five minutes from your office"—he was in Towson—" so you can either put him on the phone, or I'm going into his office, I don't care if you've got twenty armed guards in front of me, I'm getting in his office or I'm going to be loud enough to where he can hear me, and trust me, I can get loud."

You don't have to do that, the assistant said.

"My husband has been sick for years now," Carol said. "He's been in the hospital for the last four months. His stomach is wide open and his guts are hanging out. His only chance is to go to Cleveland *tonight*. They're ready for us. The judge has declared him disabled, but Medicaid will not take effect for forty-five more days. In forty-five days, my husband will be dead."

The assistant took Gary's name and details.

Give me ten minutes, the assistant said. I will call you back.

Carol sat in her car by the side of the road, waiting. Cars whisked by. Five minutes passed, and her phone rang. It was Congressman Robert Zirkin, who said, Mrs. Stern, I understand what you're going through, and I'm going to help you.

# 66

Congressman Zirkin asked Carol which social security office Carol was closest to.

"Reisterstown," Carol said.

"Go to the Social Security office in Owings Mills, and go up to the officer and give him your name. I'm going to make a call. Can you head over there now?"

"You just helped to save my husband's life," Carol said.

She turned around.

"I was at the social security office in about ten minutes," Carol said.

When she gave the guard her name, he told her to follow him, which she did, along a hallway to two desks. When Carol gave her name again, one of the two women at the desks—who was wearing a suit—indicated she was ready for Carol.

She'll take good care of you, the guard said. I hope your husband will be okay.

What can I do for you? The woman in the suit asked.

"Can you call the woman at Dr. Kareem's office at the Cleveland Clinic?" Carol asked. "And then fax everything showing that Gary has Medicare, and he is fully covered, and he is ready to go. Ask her if she needs anything else and let her know that my husband has Medicaid."

No problem, she said, then left and shortly returned. Your husband is all set, she told Carol. I faxed over everything they need from us, and she told me to let you know you only need to call if you have any questions.

Carol started driving back to the motor vehicles office to get her license.

"And I'm almost three-quarters of the way there," Carol said, "when I get another phone call that said, We've got another problem. Okay," I said, "what's this problem? They said that it's a lateral move. I'm like, Yeah? What the hell is a lateral move? From one hospital to another?"

"They won't pay for a lateral move," Carol said, "which means you have to drive him there. I'm like, Gary will be dead if I drive him there, he has to be helicoptered there, or jetted there, and . . ."

"They said," David later explained, "they would drive him in an ambulance."

I said, "And bounce him up and down the road the whole way there."

"It wasn't an option," Carol said. "There was no way he could make it; he would be dead before he got there."

"I'll call you back," Carol said.

Carol hung up the phone.

Carol was heading along a long road out in Westminster County when she saw a big sign: NEED MEDICAL TRANSPORT? With a telephone number.

Medical transport?

Air transport?

That's just what Gary and Carol needed. She wrote the telephone number down.

# 67

---

Carol had her new driver's license, and her new social security card with her name, Carol Bishop-Stern, on it. She was all set—except she didn't have the money to pay for the medical jet.

"I explained to the medical transport company what's going on," Carol said. "They said they could reroute a plane and have it there by tonight and it would cost $10,500, half of the normal cost, so I said okay."

She needed to get a cashiers' check for $10,500, plus paperwork signed by a notary to give to the pilot. She also needed a doctor to call the University of Maryland Hospital to write orders for transport.

She called Lee Weith, her Wells Fargo banker in Baltimore, and said, "I need you to call this number and find out what they need. I need a cashier's check. Please take out $10,500 from my savings account."

She had about $15,000 in it from a previous settled workman's comp case. Carol told her banker to take everything, every penny, if they had to.

She called the medical transport service back and said, "It's a go."

Carol went to the bank. Lee had the papers ready to sign.

Carol made it back to the house by 1:00. She had half an hour to pack. David came by to the house while Carol was tossing stuff in a suitcase.

"We're going to be leaving between 6:00 and 7:00 o'clock tonight," Carol told him. "Everything is a go with the Cleveland Clinic."

Dr. Kareem would meet them the following morning, Saturday, at about eight o'clock.

While David was driving her to the hospital to pick up Gary, Carol got a call from the medical transport company letting her know they were rerouting a plane and would be picking them up at 6:30.

Carol prayed, "God, angels, Jesus, thank you, my husband's going to live. And it's only because you pointed me in the right direction" with the medical transport sign. "Gary's going to live. And not only is he going to live, they're giving him new intestines. He's going to have a whole new life. We're going to have our life back."

# 68

---

On WB5, the entire staff was somber. Everyone had been told Gary was going home on hospice, going home to die. Only Gary's doctors and Sunny knew about Cleveland. But, as the news about the Cleveland Clinic spread, everyone was excited about Gary's last chance.

"Instead of preparing for a funeral," Carol said, "they had a celebration in Gary's room."

Doctors, nurses, LPN's, security guards, attendants, general staff, including the clean-up crew, were showing up with smiles for Gary to wish him luck.

A little after 6:00 in the evening, a staff of eight, all dressed in flight gear, came up to Gary's room

"It looked as if they were coming to pick up some sort of dignitary," one of the nurses told Carol. "This has never happened here before, but we've never had someone like you and Gary here before."

"But Sunny wasn't there," Carol said.

Sunny always worked the night shift, and she hadn't come in yet. They went downstairs, where there were two ambulances waiting to take them to the airport. One of the drivers got a phone call, saying we had to wait for about five minutes. Sunny came running out the door, saying, "You can't leave without saying good-bye."

Everyone was being careful with Gary, but Carol knew she had not brought her husband this far for him to die. "He will not overdose on medications, so, if he needs pain killers, give it to him."

Dr. Chun said, <u>She's absolutely right, I will write the orders for it . . .</u>

When Gary left the University of Maryland Hospital, the nurses lined up to say good-bye.

"Even the ones that Gary had yelled at," Carol said. "And they all wished him luck, and they all said they loved him."

Now Gary was laughing and joking about how he's going to eat crabs again, how he's going to eat *everything* again, how he was going to dance with his wife again.

The Texas Stomp.

At the Cantina.

Carol was speechless. Unusual for her.

Dr. Chun asked if they could go into the hall, one last time.

How did you do it? Dr. Chun asked.

"How did I do what?" Carol asked.

How did you manage to get him Medicaid and how did you manage to get medical transportation?

"Dr. Chun," Carol said, "don't you know me by now?"

Dr. Chun smiled and said, Yes, I do.

"I accomplished something that day that made me feel proud," Carol said.

## 69

"How do I describe the flight to Cleveland?" Carol said.

Gary was terrified, but also felt as if he had a second chance. At the Baltimore-Washington International Airport, the ambulance drove them to the area where the private jets were. Even though the flight was only an hour, the flight nurse made sure Gary—who was lying next to a window—was comfortable.

During the flight, Gary kept smiling at Carol and telling her he loved her.

## 70

Carol had never been in Cleveland before. The only things she knew about the city: the Browns and snow.

The Clinic is over one hundred and fifty acres. It has about forty buildings, including three hotels, so big it has its own zip code.

"The Cleveland Clinic had never seen someone in Gary's condition before," Carol said. "The next day, which was a Saturday, the nurses were telling me that we were not going to see Dr. Kareem until Monday because he didn't come in on the weekends. I said, 'No, Dr. Kareem will be here.'"

That's never happened before, one of the nurses said.

A half hour later, Dr. Kareem came in with his entire team.

The first thing he did was introduce himself to Gary.

"Then he looked at me," Carol said, "and he said, 'Who's this?'"

"This is my angel," Gary said. "This is my wife, Carol."

Gary's right, Dr. Kareem said to Carol, you are an angel . . . My assistant told me what you did to get Gary here this weekend. How did you do that? "I'm no angel," Carol said. "But there were a lot of angels involved to get it done."

I feel like I already know you, Mr. Stern, Dr. Kareem said. I've spent hours on the phone with Dr. Chun and Dr. Cross.

"I have a question for you," Carol asked. "When you have a patient in surgery, what's the first thing you do?"

Dr. Kareem said, I say a prayer.

"Then," Carol said, "you're the right man for the job."

# 71

---

Dr. Kareem examined Gary. He tweaked the TPN. He measured every fistula. He had almost three dozen tests done. They checked Gary out from head-to-toe and cut back on his pain medication.

"Gary got scared," Carol said. "They were taking him down for a lot of tests. Gary went into a place I've never seen before. He didn't watch TV. He didn't talk. He didn't drink sips. He didn't ask for anything. He folded his arms up and just stared. He didn't sleep, he just stared. I talked to him, and it was like I wasn't even there, he didn't talk back. He didn't yell."

Carol called David and said, "I don't know what to do."

Carol asked if one of the dogs from the pediatric ward could visit Gary. Gary bent down to pet the dog, but he didn't say anything.

Carol, David, and Stacey took Gary in his wheelchair to the top of the Cleveland Clinic.

They looked north toward Canada. At night, you could see a big illuminated ferris wheel.

Gary wouldn't talk.

"He wouldn't even talk to Dr. Kareem," Carol said.

She called Dr. Chun and told him maybe the Cleveland Clinic was the wrong place.

"He stayed on the phone with me for an hour," Carol said.

You [had] this hospital wired, Dr. Chun said. You knew all the doctors, you knew where to find everybody, everybody knew you . . . [Y]ou came and went on your own, and nobody ever bothered you, because you were part of the hospital. You're just not used to this [new] hospital.

"It's not me," Carol said, "it's Gary. He's different. Are you sure Dr. Kareem is the right one?"

Carol . . . you have always trusted me, Dr. Chun said. [Y]ou've always believed in me. . . Dr. Kareem is the right man for Gary. You have to have faith.

Finally Gary began talking.

A little.

Gary started talking a little more. He talked to David about basketball.

The hospital Chapel was on the first floor, down a hall lined with paintings—Native Americans.

"It was a small Chapel," Carol said. "It had four or five rows of candles and an altar that you stepped up to. It had a cross, but Jesus wasn't on the cross. There was a picture of the Virgin Mary in the back where the candles were." The burning candles gave off the scent of incense. "And, I think Saint Peter, the patron saint of fishermen," which Carol figured would include crabs.

Carol recited the Lord's Prayer and then, as she usually did, talked to God, "asking for help and asking for strength and asking for Gary to be okay and asking *Why*, and what He needs me to do, to keep going on."

She had said "that prayer more times than I can count, because I couldn't see why God would let anyone go through what Gary went through, without it meaning something."

"I feel strongly that this is one of the main reasons Gary had to go through what he did," Carol said, "and Dave and I had to go through what we did was to help other people who were in a similar situation."

"And," Carol said, "God would tell me <u>Patience—and don't forget what you see</u>. Trust me, there's no way I can forget what I saw. There's no way I can forget the sound of my husband's voice or the fear on his face or his laughter."

Carol walked outside the Cleveland Clinic.

"They don't want you walking out there," Carol said, "because it's a bad area. I always said the same thing, 'I'm going to be fine. No one's going to hurt me, because there's a reason why I'm still here, there's a reason why I'm seeing the things that I have seen, and God's not going to want that to stop until I can tell people—be a witness—for other people in distress.'"

# 72

Dr. Kareem put off Gary's surgery a couple of times, once because Gary had an infection, and another time because of Gary's depression. Dr. Kareem wanted to make sure Gary was ready physically and psychologically before surgery.

The day finally came for what would be a sixteen-hour surgery.

David thought Dr. Kareem was a miracle worker.

Before transplanting Gary's intestine (along with his liver and other organs that would have to be replaced—a much more dangerous procedure), Dr. Kareem wanted to see if he could save Gary's intestine, to keep the intestine from developing leaky fistulas. And he wanted to make sure Gary was strong enough to take the antirejection medication.

After the surgery, when Dr. Kareem sat down with Carol, she could tell he was exhausted. He told her Gary was doing fine. He had to take all but forty-two centimeters (sixteen and a half inches) of his small intestines and half his colon. The surgical staples, which looked like a zipper, extended (as David described it) "from his cock to below his chin."

But Gary was closed.

# 73

---

Three weeks after Gary's surgery, Dr. Kareem came in to Gary's room with the pathology report, which showed Gary had no active Crohns. All Gary's fistulas were related to his earlier surgeries.

"I could of told you that," Gary said.

I'm sure you could, Dr. Kareem said. You know your body better than anyone. However, I needed the report. You will not get another fistula.

"I've heard that before," Carol said. "How can you be so sure?"

Because I did the surgery, Dr. Kareem said. Gary will not get another fistula. I will stake my reputation on it.

Dr. Kareem started Gary on clear liquids. Having any nutrition by mouth was a big deal.

"The first time I went in there and Gary was closed," Carol said, "I looked down at his abdomen and he had stiches going all the way down, and I couldn't help but think that was the sexiest man I had ever seen in my life. And it's strange. When Gary finally went to the bathroom, when it was clear everything was functioning, Carol, the nurses shouted, Carol, Gary's going to the bathroom, Gary's going to the bathroom!"

"That's when I decided to move him to the Outer Banks," Carol said. "He was still having TPN, but he could slowly start eating food."

Most people have six feet of intestines. Gary had seventeen inches.

"Food would go straight through him," Carol said.

Gary ate for the taste, the feel of eating. Gary decided he didn't want a transplant. Not now. Not yet.

"He just didn't want to go through any more operations," Carol said.

# 74

---

In the middle of June, it was time for Gary to be discharged.

Dr. Kareem wanted him to stay in Cleveland for a while so he could monitor Gary's progress.

"I knew Gary was doing better," Carol said. "I knew it was time for him to get out of the hospital, because if he stayed there, we were taking the chance of him getting an infection in his line."

Iatrogenic diseases—diseases caused by medical or surgical intervention, disease you get because you are in a hospital—are the leading cause of death in the United States—not cancer (about 565,000 deaths per year), not heart disease (about 700,000 deaths per year), but medical negligence and an environment with many potential threats (about 800,000 deaths per year, the number one cause).

According to *Death by Medicine*, a review funded by the Nutrition Institute of America, the care given to thousands of patients every year was making them sick.

A US Department of Health and Human Services report estimated one in seven hospitalized Medicare beneficiaries are harmed by the medical system. A 2014 report published in the *Journal of the American Medical Association* (JAMA) estimated up to 50 percent of all hospital deaths were connected to sepsis. Every year, seven and a half million unnecessary surgical and medical procedures are performed. Eight million nine hundred thousand people were unnecessarily hospitalized.

The Centers for Disease Control estimate tens of millions of unnecessary antibiotics are prescribed for viral infections. Every year, one hundred six thousand deaths are caused by adverse drug reactions. Two hundred three thousand deaths are caused by bed sores and infection. The total number of iatrogenic deaths is 783,936 annually. Since only 20 percent of adverse iatrogenic events are reported, the number might be higher.

Gary and Carol had planned to go to the "top of the Cleveland Clinic for the Fourth of July fireworks," but Gary was having a bad day.

It didn't matter. For the first time in years, Carol was relieved. Staying near the Cleveland Clinic? No problem. They'd move to a hotel.

"The first hotel was too expensive," Carol said. "The second one was too filthy. The third one was just right."

It was the Goldilocks Hotel.

## 75

"[T]he really remarkable thing is the surgeon closed him," Dr. Chun said. "Now, he had to take a massive amount of small bowel so that [Gary] was dependent on nutrition through the vein to survive, but importantly, Gary was able to have quality of life, he was able to leave the hospital, he was able to walk around without these holes spitting out fluid on his abdomen . . ."

Dr. Kareem had performed the operation but, Dr. Chun told Carol it was Carol who had saved Gary.

Before they left Cleveland, Carol arranged for the best restaurant in the hotel to give a candlelight dinner for Gary and her on the rooftop of the hospital: crab cakes, mashed potatoes, rolls, and chocolate cake.

"It was a warm and clear night," Carol said. "So many stars. Gary and I sat up there, talking about the future, about *having* a future."

They discussed moving to the Outer Banks of North Carolina, where, on their first trip to Ocean City they had watched the dolphins swim past.

Carol liked the idea.

They talked about walking on the beach, about watching the dogs play and run, about Gary catching his own crabs, about watching Jade play softball, watching her in a school play. . .

"For a short time," Carol said, "Gary and I had our lives back."

# 76

They had been going to Dr. Kareem's office twice a week. The last time they saw him, Dr. Kareem told Gary, I don't need to see you for two months.

Gary looked at Carol and said, "We can go home."

You are a perfect candidate for an intestinal transplant, Dr. Kareem said. However, you need to get stronger now, both physically and psychologically.

That was Gary's job.

For a transplant—and now Gary was willing to consider it—Gary had to get off the TPN and be able to handle the anti-rejection medication.

Going home.

"But," Carol said, "I couldn't just get on a regular plane with Gary."

Insurance wouldn't pay for the flight back in a medical transport.

"And I couldn't just rent a car," Carol said. "What if Gary had a seizure?"

She needed to have all of his medical supplies with them.

Once again, she called Kenny. Once again, Kenny left his job and rented an RV, which he had professionally sterilized. It had a bathroom, a bedroom, a living room, and a kitchen.

"Kenny bought sheets, washed them," Carol said, "bought blankets, washed them, pillow cases, washed them, pillows—everything was brand new."

Kenny stocked the RV's refrigerator with Gary's favorite drinks and put in a supply of Gary's favorite snacks, including some they could cook on the RV stove, or in the van microwave.

Kenny and Jade pulled up to the hotel on July 6th. He had forgotten it was the Fourth of July weekend. Carol got Gary into his wheelchair and brought him down to the van.

"When Kenny helped him up the stairs into the van, Gary looked around," Carol said. "It was like the old Gary was coming back."

"Hey," Gary said about the RV, "we have got to buy one of these. Let's make a long trip out of it. Gee, I wish David had come."

The first forty-five minutes going home were rough for Gary. The roads in Cleveland were in bad shape. Once they hit the open road, Gary—on the bed—sang out, "Dairy Queen. Dairy Queen." It took Carol and Kenny a couple of minutes to realize what he was saying. They stopped at the first Dairy Queen they came to. Gary and Jade had hot fudge sundaes.

"Now," Carol said, "this might not seem like much to anyone else, but Gary eating a hot fudge sundae meant everything to us."

"We sat in the Dairy Queen for at least an hour," Carol said, "maybe an hour and a half."

And Gary did not get sick or go to the bathroom.

"Food was staying in his system a little bit longer," Carol said.

They called David and Stacey and let them know when they were going to arrive in Baltimore. David was waiting with Stacey and Butchy when they pulled up. Barbara and her son Chuck came over that night.

Gary was allowed to eat whatever he wanted at this point, but he was supposed to be eating in moderation, only four to six ounces at a time, let it settle, wait an hour, and then eat again.

"But this is Gary, right?" Carol said. "I would remind him, 'Gary, remember, you're not supposed to eat so much,'" Carol said. "But I wasn't going to be a nag at this point."

Gary didn't have a lot of pleasures left.

## 77

The next day, they arrived in Baltimore, the first time Gary had been home in over seven months. Carol and Kenny had made a lot of changes to the house to make life easier for Gary. The only dog there was Butchy. Zenny and Princie were already in North Carolina.

Carol needed to 1) make Gary's doctor appointments, 2) arrange for a nurse to come every week, 3) arrange for the Equinox deliveries of medication and TPN, 4) find doctors in North Carolina, 5) put the Baltimore house on the market, and 6) find a place to live in North Carolina.

Kenny, with help from his friend DJ, needed to finish the rest of the house, so they could sell it before the bank foreclosed.

David had to work. Because he and Stacey had been taking a lot of time off, they didn't have as much money flowing in.

"They were giving us more money than they could afford," Carol said, "but they never told me that."

Carol's mom, Jeanette, and her sister Linda and their church in West Virginia "also helped us out again."

"We all knew Gary was going to keep going back and forth to the hospital," Carol said.

Kenny went back to North Carolina to look for a place he could afford without a job and big enough for Gary's and Carol's things, including three dogs and Kenny's cat. He found one on Waterlily Street in Currituck County. Kenny moved everything to the new house except Butchy, who stayed with Gary until he and Carol moved.

# 78

Gary and Carol and Butchy were driving from Baltimore to Waterlily Street in a van that had been fitted out as an ambulance with a PortaPotty.

"The ride was too much for Gary," Carol said. "Two hours into the trip, Butchy started running from the back of the van to the front and crying. I knew what this meant so I pulled over as Gary had a Grand Mal seizure.

Carol gave Gary his seizure medication. Half-an-hour later, they were again on their way.

Gary went to sleep and Butchy stayed on the bed with him for the rest of the trip.

"Whenever Butchy alerted me that Gary was about to have a seizure," Carol said, "he looked so proud."

Once they arrived at the Waterlily house, Gary, exhausted from the trip, stayed in bed for three days, too weak to sit up. When Gary had the strength to get up, Carol walked him to the back door, where Gary watched Zenny and Princie tearing around the backyard, which they couldn't do in Baltimore.

Gary had never seen them running free. He felt as if they were his spirit—after all the years in hospitals, after all the operations, Gary was also running free.

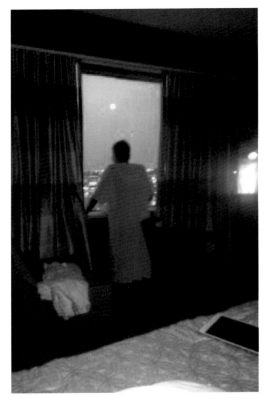

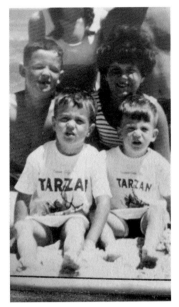

Gary Stern looks out his
hospital window, 2015.

Top: Stevie and Barbara.
Bottom: Gary and David
Stern, 1966.

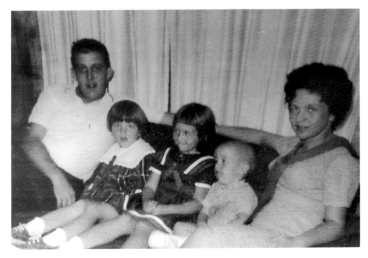

Kenneth, Kendra, Carol, Kevin, and Jeanette Bishop, 1966.

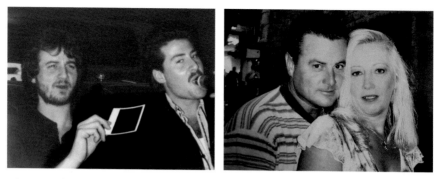

Gary and David at Doc's Bar, 1987.    Gary and Carol, 2002.

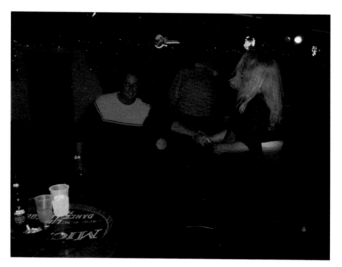

Gary and Carol, 2002.

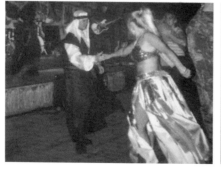

Gary and Carol
at the Cantina, 2003.

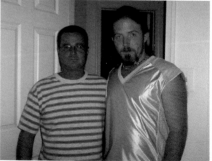

Gary and stepson Kenneth
Laughlin, 2005.

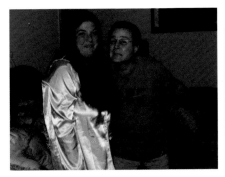

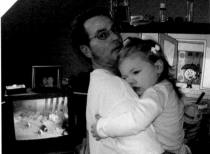

Gary and stepdaughter Kimberly
Romero, 2005.

Gary and Jade Laughlin
(granddaughter), 2007.

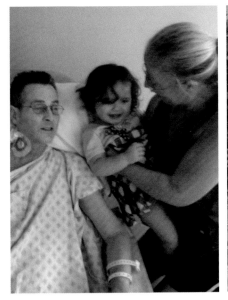

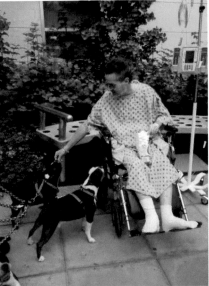

Gary meets Nadilla
(granddaughter), 2011.

Gary sees his dogs at the
hospital, 2011.

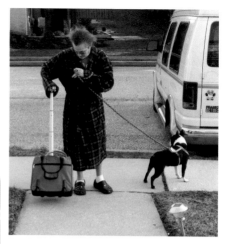

Gary comes home, September 2011.

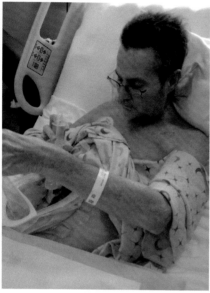

Gary cleans his fistula bag, 2011.

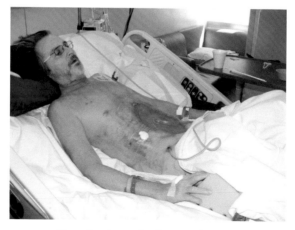

Gary back in the hospital, 2012.

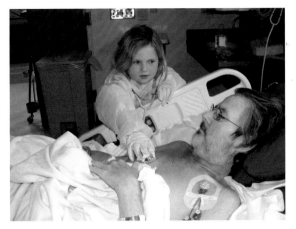

Jade trying to cheer up Gary (her Pop Pop), 2012.

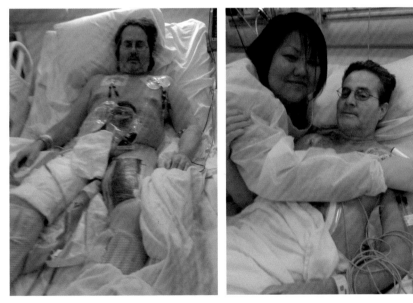

Gary's abdomen, 2012.

Gary with Sunny, his favorite
nurse at UMD, 2013.

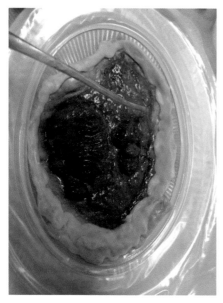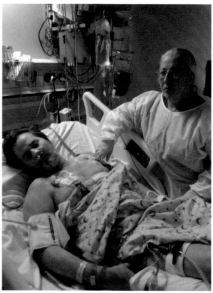

Gary at UMD with fourteen       Gary and Carol after Gary had
fistulas, 2013.                  another surgery, 2013.

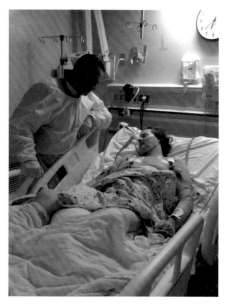

Gary and David after Gary's
surgery, 2013.

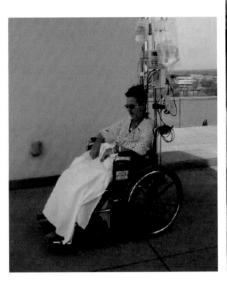

Gary at Cleveland Clinic, 2013.

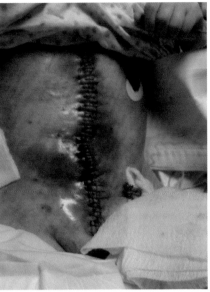

Gary closed, 2013.

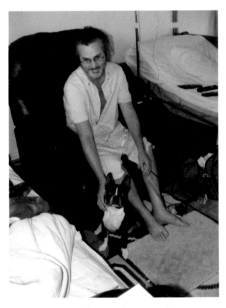

Gary with Butchy watching
for seizures, 2014.

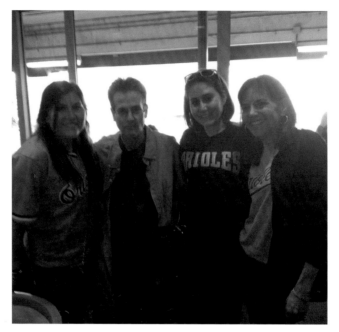

Taylor, Gary, Shannon, and Stacey at an
Orioles game, 2015.

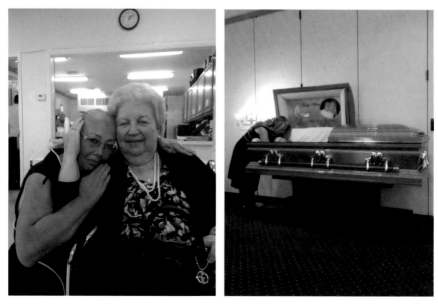

Carol and Jeanette
(Carol's mom), 2016.

Carol saying good-bye
to Gary, 2016.

"This is the life we've been looking for," Gary told Carol

Gary was as calm and relaxed as Carol had ever seen.

That same day was the first time Gary used the bidet Carol had installed in the bathroom. He loved it. He could clean himself. Independence.

# 79

Carol and Kenny took Gary to the beach.

"Kenny took one side of Gary," Carol said, "and I took the other side,"

The three of them staggered like Gary's Stooges down Avalon Pier, where he saw the dolphins in the water.

"I want my feet in the sand," Gary said.

Carol and Kenny took him to the water's edge.

"Do you want me to carry you?" Kenny asked.

"I want to walk," Gary said.

As he waded in, he said, "Look, Carol, a seashell."

Half an oyster shell.

Kenny picked it up and put it in his pocket.

"Don't worry, Pop-pop," he said, "I'll make sure we bring it back with us."

They took Gary back to the van and washed the sand off his feet.

"I think I'm ready to go home now," Gary said.

Carol still has the shell.

# 80

One afternoon at home, "Gary ate at least a dozen crabs," Carol said. "Maybe eighteen."

Kenny weighs two thirty, and he couldn't keep up with Gary.

"But here's the sad thing," Carol said. "Gary would have a trash bag next to him. He'd eat the crabs and get sick. Then he would go back to eating them again."

Gary wanted to buy crabs in bulk. It was cheaper. He investigated buying a refrigerated truck for all the crabs.

"North Carolina is a great place to live," Carol said. "They move in two speeds: slow and gone fishing."

When they lived on Waterlily, the first doctor with whom they had an appointment left a sign on his locked door: "Beautiful day. I went home to cut the grass, and I'm going fishing."

"It was like Mayberry RFD," Carol said.

In fact, Andy Griffith had a place nearby in Manteo.

To give Gary some of his independence, Carol got him a rider-mower. He would have preferred a Corvette. A red one.

Gary liked the Outer Banks. He liked the drive-through beer shops like the Brew Thru. He liked the Zip Lines. He liked the limit on how high people could build. He liked having the sound on one side of their island and the beach on the other.

Gary liked the South Border coffee shop. Gary liked the Sugar Creek Seafood Restaurant, which was right on the water—even over the water. Gary liked another restaurant called Barefoot Bernie's; the food was good and they gave a lot of work to people with autism. Gary liked the Food Lion supermarkets and Harris Teeter, where Carol bought lamb chops, which she steam-baked. Gary liked the islands' names, like Nags Head and Kill Devil Hills. Gary liked the miniature golf and the Go-Karts. Gary liked the salt-water taffy. Gary liked that you could find buried arrowheads. Off of Mile Post 6, legend has it that Blackbeard's ship went aground. Maybe more than one ship.

"They say that from a helicopter you can see three of Blackbeard's sunken ships," Carol said. "They say he buried treasure somewhere on the islands."

Gary liked that Blackbeard spent time in the area.

Gary liked that you could fish off the bridges. Gary liked the charter fishing. Gary liked whale watching. Gary liked parasailing. Gary liked Beach Road, where—before he got sick—he and Carol would sit in the car, watch the waves, and eat lunch. Gary liked the peace.

When Gary and Carol took Robert, Carol's ex-husband, to dinner, Robert could tell Gary was sicker than he'd thought. He was shocked by how much weight Gary had lost.

"Half his body weight," Robert estimated.

Often, Carol went to Robert for moral support. She went to him to cry because she didn't want to cry at home in front of Gary. She borrowed money from Robert.

"She was living paycheck to paycheck," Robert said.

Occasionally, Carol read to Gary or they would watch a superhero movie together.

"*Wolverine,*" Carol said. "We watched a lot of *Big Brother*—he loved that. *Survivor*, too." Of course, because Gary was a survivor.

Jade was, of course, a Ravens fan.

"When she was a year old, she got her very first cheerleading outfit," Carol said. "For the Ravens." To Jade, Carol said, "Pop-Pop picked that out. You remember that pink horse? Pop-Pop picked that out, too."

"It had sparkly hair," Jade said. "It was like a rocking horse."

"He loved picking things out for you," Carol said. "He got you a lot of books that you guys read together."

"Princess books," Jade said. "*Beauty and the Beast*, 'Aurora.' I used to call her Sleeping Beauty. I couldn't say beauty, so whenever I said beauty it sounded like buddy. I sounded like I was from New Jersey. Hmm."

Gary went to Jade's softball games.

"I would be catcher, and I would be, like, second choice for the outfield," Jade said. "I always caught the ball."

Jade also remembered a crab-eating contest with Gary.

"We had to see who could eat them the fastest," Jade said. "Without messing up or hurting ourselves. We didn't have any choice about hurting ourselves, because, of course, [the shells are] going to be sharp when you break [them] off. You don't want to cut your gums or your lips, which I did a lot."

Jade's record was "six, seven, eight?" Jade guessed. "Ten?"

Gary never used a hammer to crack the claws—he disdained using a hammer—he used the back of his knife.

# 81

For Thanksgiving, Kimberly and Nadilla, then 4 years old, came from California.

Nadilla hadn't seen them for over two years. Carol and Kimberly worried about Nadilla getting excited and hitting Gary's stomach. But on the first day, they realized they were worrying for nothing. Nadilla got up on the bed with her Paw-Paw.

"Paw-Paw," Nadilla asked, "why?"

"Why what?" Gary asked.

Nadilla pointed at his stomach.

"Why does my tummy look like this?" Gary said.

Nadilla shook her head yes.

Gary thought about it for a second or two and then said, "because I got too hungry, and I swallowed a ball."

"I don't get that hungry," Nadilla said.

"No," Gary said, "don't do that."

The next day Carol made donuts with the grandkids—Jade, Logan, and Nadilla. Eating donuts. Not the medical kind.

Nadilla got upset.

"She didn't want Paw-Paw to have the plate of donuts," Carol said, "until we took the donut holes off the plate."

She said. "Paw-Paw can't eat balls."

That afternoon, they played softball. Kenny moved Gary's bed and opened the window so Gary could be a part of the game.

"I explained to her that when it comes to Pop-Pop, you have to be easy," Carol said. "You have to be clean."

When she was going to Gary, Nadilla washed her hands, sanitized them, put on gloves, and put on a safety garment, so nothing she touched could transfer an infection.

Jade would check Gary's vitals, check his sugar, and she would write it down.

"She would help me with his TPN," Carol said.

When she finished taking care of Gary, Gary would help her with her homework.

She never asked about death.

# 82

The North Carolina doctors were spread out. The pain doctor was an hour away in Virginia, and the GI Doctor was two hours away in Greenville. It was hard to get Gary to Greenville and back in one day.

The dietitian was also two hours away in Greenville. Gary's primary doctor was forty-five minutes away in the Outer Banks.

"I was having trouble getting them to talk to each other," Carol said.

"Gary would have a seizure," Carol said. "One doctor would want to start Gary on one medication, and I would have to call all the others to make sure they knew—and agreed."

An occasional workman at the house knew about Gary's condition. He was pulling up to the house when Gary had a Grand Mal seizure. Carol called 911. As Gary was being put in the ambulance, Carol was putting Gary's medication in the cabinet. They were gone for five hours. The morning after they got home, Carol went to get Gary's pain medication, and a hundred and twenty ounces of liquid Dilaudid was gone; half of Gary's medication.

"I wanted to beat the shit out of that guy" Carol said, "but first I needed to get Gary some more medication. And that's not easy."

Carol got a little more Dilaudid, but it wasn't enough.

"Thank God for marijuana," Carol said.

Gary's pain management doctor did a urinalysis on his next visit, and Gary tested positive, a problem, which influenced Gary's pain doctor, who (like other previous doctors) worried Gary was getting dependent on drugs. Marijuana was helping more than anything else with Gary's pain and his seizures.

While Carol was trying to get his medication, Gary was sinking into depression.

Often, Carol stayed up for three and four days straight. When she finally slept, it was only a cat nap. That schedule went on for five weeks, when Carol ended up in the hospital for exhaustion.

Kenny took over caring for Gary, which meant yet again he had to take some time off from his job at Exotic Homes.

When Kenny picked them up from the hospital, Gary looked great.

"Two weeks after I got out of the hospital," Carol said, "I ran into the guy who took Gary's medication at a Hardee's restaurant."

He was in the front passenger seat of his truck. Carol parked her van and walked to the truck.

"Look, you SOB," Carol said, "you stole my husband's medication. Get out of that truck. I'm going to kick your ass. No one fucks with my husband."

The workman played stupid. And he wouldn't get out of the truck.

Because Gary needed more painkillers than the doctors felt comfortable giving him, Carol had to find another pain management doctor, which was harder than she expected.

# 83

Because Gary was having a good day, Carol decided to tell him some of the things she had kept from him, things that could have, under other conditions, driven Gary to despair, like the times the doctors were saying that Gary wasn't going to make it and that Carol should call the family to say good-bye.

Gary nodded as he listened. He knew more than Carol suspected.

"You heard what Dr. Cross said about the fistulas not coming from Crohn's?" Gary asked David. "It means I was right all along. I kept telling everyone it wasn't my Crohn's, and no one would believe me."

"Babe," Carol said, "I did."

"The doctors didn't."

"The Doctors at UMD did."

"They weren't the ones who fucked me up," Gary had said.

"Do you think we should sue?" David asked.

"Hell, yes," Gary said.

# Part Three

---

# Heart of a Mule

# 84

Gary and Carol had talked about a lawsuit from day one, but it never seemed important to focus on. Getting Gary healthy was the focus. But now, Gary decided he wanted to fight back, to sue for malpractice, to get enough money to take care of Carol for the rest of her life. Carol wanted money from a lawsuit to cover Gary's needs.

They contacted Peter Angelos's office—Angelos was the best law firm in Baltimore, probably in Maryland. She thought the name was a good omen: *Angelos-angels.*

Angelos—whose family, Greek immigrants, moved to Baltimore when he was ten—grew grew up in tough circumstances. His father, John, immigrated from Μενετές Καρπάθου, Karpathos, Greece to the United States. He married Georgia Kousouris in 1966, and they had two children, John and Louis. They settled in the working-class neighborhood of Highlandtown, and lived in a row house. Angelos's father owned a local tavern, where Peter worked as a young man. At home, they mostly spoke Greek.

Because of the neighborhood, Angelos learned how to box.

On the internet, the firm is described as "synonymous with service—and success. As an attorney for more than fifty years, he has devoted his professional life to representing those who have suffered from abuse by clergy, exposure to harmful asbestos fibers, defective products, medical malpractice, and personal injury. Peter Angelos is a passionate advocate and a tireless champion for Baltimore, his hometown."

Angelos, a graduate of the Eastern College of Commerce and Law and the University of Baltimore School of Law, where he was class valedictorian, was among the first attorneys in the country to litigate asbestos cases and childhood lead-poisoning cases. He took on the tobacco industry. And he has represented the Maryland Building and Construction Trades councils, the Steelworkers' unions, and other labor organizations. The AFL-CIO gave him its Social Justice Award. Among many other honors, he has received the

Ellis Island Medal of Honor Society and has been honored by the Associated Black Charities of Maryland. Angelos has consistently championed the underdog, "survivors and victims"—steelworkers, shipyard workers, veterans suffering from various disabilities—a good sign, Carol thought.

Another good sign: Angelos organized a group to buy the Baltimore Orioles so the team could stay in Baltimore.

He also bred racehorses, an interest he shared with Gary.

The firm took Gary's case, which was assigned to Thomas C. Summers, a graduate of Dickenson College and the University of Baltimore School of Law and the head of Angelos's medical malpractice group, who had tried over one hundred medical malpractice-personal injury cases.

The case might be difficult. It was sure to be expensive.

When he called Carol at the Cleveland Clinic, he asked, <u>Do you really think we have a case?</u>

<u>What are you talking about?</u> Carol said. "I know we have a case. I'm positive of it. I've had conversations with several doctors, and all of them told me the same thing. They weren't going to name names, because doctors don't do that, but they believed there were screw-ups."

<u>I hate to bring it up</u>, Summers said, and he reminded Carol that if Gary died, he'd have to have an autopsy, which would be problematic because Judaism had prohibitions against autopsies and, without an autopsy that could help pin down what had caused Gary's condition, they were at a disadvantage.

But after Dr. Kareem operated on Gary and gave Gary a short gut, he told Carol that he sent his intestines off to pathology.

"Why?" Carol asked.

<u>I need to know if Gary had active Crohn's</u>, Dr. Kareem said, <u>just in case he needs medication for Crohn's Disease.</u>

When the pathology report came back, Dr. Kareem told Carol he had good news for her. He told Carol there was no active Crohn's, nor had there been any active Crohn's when Gary first went into the hospital. According to Dr. Kareem, the Crohn's looked like it had been dormant for about ten years.

"God made it so that Gary could have an autopsy done of his intestines," Carol said, "while Gary was still alive."

Carol called Tom Summers and said, "You wanted an autopsy, well, you got your autopsy, and I still have my husband. Dr. Kareem managed to do an autopsy on Gary's intestines while Gary was still alive."

She told Summers about the pathology report done on the intestines and about how all the fistulas had been related to the previous surgeries.

Summers asked for a copy of the report, which Carol faxed.

## 85

When Summers moved to another firm, Gary's case was taken over by Jay Miller, who also had impressive credentials: a BA from the University of Baltimore, who would be listed in the Bar Register of Pre-eminent Lawyers, among the Top 100 Trial Lawyers by National Trial Lawyers, and as a Super Lawyer in Maryland Super Lawyers Magazine.

At the beginning, Miller said he "wasn't interested in the story. I was interested in [it] from a very legal standpoint: was he in a wheelchair, being fed through a tube, because of something some doctor or combination of doctors did wrong? And that was a very difficult process for them, because that took some time, you know? [Gary] had a complicated medical history."

Miller said, "Look, why don't you bring him down here, let me meet with him, let me meet with the both of you, and let's see if this is a case we can get ready for trial."

"I can't bring [Gary] to Baltimore," Carol said. "My van is broken down. And I have no money."

"How much do you need?" Miller asked.

"I can't ask you for money," Carol said. "It's not allowed."

"It won't be coming from the firm," Miller continued. "I will give it to you for my own pocket."

"I've never done it before," Miller said, "but I wanted to do it for this lady to get her husband here. So I sent them whatever it was, and it wasn't a ton of money . . . because there was just something about them."

Carol got the van fixed.

Kenny had gotten the van converted at Beach Ready Auto Care to fit Gary's needs. It had a hook for Gary's emergency bag, a bed, and a toilet.

She drove Gary to Baltimore to meet Miller.

After the conference, Miller asked, "What else can I do for you while you're here?"

"What about the Orioles?" Carol asked.

Carol knew Miller's boss, Peter Angelos, owned the Orioles.

"We . . . made sure they"—including Shannon and Taylor, Barbara and Chuck—"got to an Orioles game that night with Skybox seating because of [Gary's] wheelchair," Miller said.

"Gary even had his own waitress," Carol said. "He was treated like a king. The way it should be. Gary wanted to fight, again."

"After that [Carol] thought I could do no wrong, because I was treating them like human beings, and they hadn't felt that before. That's all that lady wanted. That's all either one of them wanted . . . They were no longer just a case, they were being treated like people. It's easier for us as trial lawyers to tell a story, but to tell the story, you've got to hear the story. How do you hear the story? You've got to meet the client, you've got to talk to them, and you've got to listen."

Gary and Carol liked him immediately.

Miller arranged for a video, "A Day In The Life Of Gary Stern," which displayed the horrible condition Gary had been in.

Once it was clear to Miller "that a simple endoscopy would have discovered the bleeding ulcer," he figured they had a good case.

Miller's opinion was that instead of treating the ulcer, the doctors "went in assuming that [Gary] had a flare of Crohn's and they wanted to remove the part of the bowel that had Crohn's . . . and that set off this cascading of events where he kept having surgery after surgery on his bowels . . . Carol made it very difficult for me to say no, because she doesn't take no for an answer. And you know, the more I would tell her how difficult the case was going to be, and maybe we could try to settle, the more she would say, 'No, you're his, this is your job now. It's time for you to fight this part, I'm keeping him healthy and happy, and alive, and now you need to fight for him.' I drank the Kool-Aid because . . . I saw what she was doing for this guy, which I had never seen before, and I've been doing this [for] thirty years, I had never seen a woman really dedicate her life in such a fashion that she did to take care of him. So, that's when I started to learn the story, and it really was sort of an act of love on her part. . . [I]t wasn't that he wanted to prove that somebody did him wrong, he wanted to get what was coming to him, so Carol would be taken care of . . ." Carol "had taken such good care of him that . . . he wanted to take care of her. Because he was a man's man . . . he didn't like being helpless, believe me. Hated it."

Even during the trial, Miller thought they proved to be "an extraordinary couple, and it made people want to help . . . Even the porter at the hotel where they stayed during the trial, when he recognized Carol, he just beamed . . . [W]hatever charisma, or magic they had, I think it had to do with . . . the love they had for each other really captured people, and that's very rare, as you know."

"Well, Carol," Miller said, "that's what this trial has to be about. We've got to get you help because you're wearing down physically . . . That . . . became the theme of the trial: *If we don't get him some help, he's going to lose her because literally it was taking its toll on her physically and emotionally.*"

"Gary had lost so much with everything that had happened," Carol said. "Here's a great man who ran his own business, never slowed down, and his greatest joy in life was taking care of me. (I don't know how I ever deserved Gary.) And now he can't eat, he can't sneeze without going to the bathroom in his pants, he once owned a four-story townhouse, and now he was living in a seven-hundred-square-foot two bedroom. . . But somehow Miller managed to get Gary excited again."

Miller gave Gary the will to live again. The belief that living could be more than suffering.

# 86

Gary and Carol ran out of all their money. Kenny had to stop working to help at home, so he didn't have a paycheck coming in. He found them a smaller place. On Pinch Gut Road.

"Pinch Gut," Carol said. "Given how little intestine Gary had left, it couldn't have been more perfectly named."

"I don't want any more surgeries," Gary said. "I'm tired. I'm tired of getting sick. I'm tired of hurting. And I'm tired of seeing Carol go through this."

"I'm not going through anything I can't handle," Carol said.

"Yeah," Gary said, "that's why you were put in the hospital for exhaustion. I'm killing my wife."

"I just needed some sleep," Carol said.

## 87

Kenny helped drive Gary and Carol to West Virginia to spend a few days with Jeanette and Willem. While there, Gary always slept in a rocking chair.

"I would sleep on the couch," Carol said.

One night, after Jeanette had gone to bed, Carol and Willem watched Gary sleeping in the chair. Shrunken. Reduced.

Jeanette had said, "I need time alone with my son-in-law."

Because of her problem walking, Jeanette got around on a handicap-scooter, like a motorized wheelchair.

"She would fly on that," Carol said. "She could haul."

Carol and Willem left Jeanette and Gary alone.

If Gary asked Carol questions about Jesus, she would answer them. If he asked questions about being Catholic, about Carol's rosary, or confessions, Carol would answer. But she never pushed her religion on Gary.

"I go to churches when no one else is there," Carol explained, "because I want to fully feel my time with the Virgin Mary, Jesus, God, or one of the saints."

Carol didn't know what Jeanette said to Gary, "but," Carol said, "when they came out Gary had accepted Jesus Christ as his Lord and Savior."

Gary wanted to get baptized, but—Carol said—"he couldn't be drenched because of his central line."

# 88

---

Gary and Carol got to Baltimore a little less than two weeks before the trial. They met Miller and wanted to spend some time with David and Barbara.

They stayed at the Sheraton Inner Harbor Hotel, which had beige walls decorated with pictures, including a turn-of-the-last-century woman in an extravagant hat and a silhouette cutting of a face. There was a view of the harbor, which included a building across the way with a huge guitar on the roof.

"We finally had some money," Carol said, "so I was going to treat Gary like a king. I made sure we had two adjoining rooms and access to the VIP club house."

"Gary was up here early in the morning," said the woman who manned the club. "Always pleasant with a joke or two."

Carol made arrangements to have Gary's TPN and supplies delivered to the hotel.

When David came to spend time with Gary, Carol ducked out to get errands done. Once in a long while, Carol and David took Gary to the inner harbor to look around and sit. Occasionally, they'd go to one of the Hooters or one of the other nearby restaurants.

Gary loved to stand at the hotel room window, gaze at the ships, and talk about a future with no more doctors, no more hospitals.

"Gary didn't want anyone catering to him," Carol said, "but he wanted everyone to cater to me."

# 89

---

Gary and Carol were only ten blocks from the University of Maryland Hospital.

Gary needed his blood drawn, so Carol took him over.

"It was kind of funny," Carol said. "UMD is a big hospital, but as soon as we walked in Dr. Patel was right there. I called her name. She turned around and beamed when she saw Gary walking on his own."

"Gary you look great," Dr. Patel said.

"He's eating now." Carol said.

Dr. Chun walked up. They hadn't seen Dr. Chun since they went to Cleveland.

Dr. Chun also said Gary looked great.

"Gary lifted up his tee shirt to show me that his abdomen was closed," Dr. Chun said. "He was smiling, and quite happy. They were both happy."

Dr. Chun was not happy about their decision to move to North Carolina.

"It sounds dreamlike and great," Dr. Chun said, "but . . . as far as access to medical care . . . there's . . . big distances there to get to major medical centers. And Gary is pretty complicated, so you know, he needed to be around a center that has resources to care for complicated people, so we were obviously nervous for him."

What are you two doing here? Dr. Chun asked.

"We came for a visit," Gary said.

When are you going to have the transplant? Dr. Chun asked.

"I'm not sure," Gary said. Will you let me know? Dr. Chun said.

"I will," Carol said.

Before Dr. Patel left, Carol got a group picture of them all.

"Thank you both for everything you did for us," Gary said.

Us, not me. Still 50/50.

# 90

The trial started on a sunny and pleasant August day.

"The first day of the trial, we were ready," Carol said. "Gary and I had talked so much about it, we both knew it was going to be hard, and I needed to make sure Gary was all right."

Carol was trying to reduce the kinds of stress that could trigger a seizure.

She made a courthouse emergency bag, things she needed to bring with her every day: two changes of clothes for Gary, a small blanket, ten saline flushes, a centerline changing kit, hemostats, seizure medication, wet wipes, extra 9-volt batteries, IV tubing, central line caps, gloves, alcohol swabs, other IV medication, protonics (which can reduce acid reflux), Promethazine (which can alleviate nausea and vomiting after surgery and to prevent motion sickness but which can also reduce white blood cell production), and Gary's throw-up bucket.

"Jay had called us the night before to let us know the first day of trial would be selecting a jury," Carol said, "and someone would be picking us up that morning for court at 8:30."

Carol was up at five. Gary came out of the bathroom, calling, "Carol, are you up?"

"Do you need some medicine?" Carol asked.

"No, not yet," Gary said. "I'm worried about court today."

"This is what we've been waiting for," Carol said.

"I'm worried I'm going to have an accident," Gary said.

"I have everything we need to take care of it in my carry-on bag," Carol said. "Are you hungry?"

"Ya, but I'm afraid to eat," Gary said.

"We have three hours before we have to go," Carol said.

"Let's go to the clubhouse," Gary said.

Together, they went to the fifteenth floor, got some food, and sat at a window overlooking the Inner Harbor.

"You okay?"

"Yes and no." Gary gazed through the window. "We've been waiting for this day for so long. What if Jay can't convince the jury? What if he puts someone on the jury that doesn't believe us? What if I have an accident? What if . . ."

"Hold on, hold on, where is this coming from?"

"I'm not sure."

"How many times have you told me we have nothing to worry about?"

"Hundreds."

"Well, all right, then. We have the truth on our side."

"And a good lawyer."

# 91

"Okay," Judge Evelyn Omega Cannon said, "why don't we call the case?"

The trial was in Room 330, Courthouse East.

"This is the case of Gary Stern, and I'm going to call it 'Gary Stern, et al versus Todd Heller . . .,' and counsel would you please identify yourselves for the record?"

"Michael Warshaw, on behalf of the plaintiffs, Carol and Gary Stern."

Warshaw was working with Miller.

"Jay Miller, of the law offices of Peter Angelos, also on behalf of the plaintiffs, Gary and Carol Stern."

"Your Honor, good morning," said Penhallegon. "John Penhallegon for Dr. Todd Heller, Dr. Stephen Epstein, and Woodholme Gastroenterology."

"Good morning, Your Honor," Penhallegon's colleague said, "Valerie Grove for the same defendants."

Back at the Sheraton Inner Harbor Hotel, Carol said, "Everyone was so nice to Gary and me. I had called them before we got there to let them know I needed special accommodations and about Gary's condition. I couldn't have asked for better treatment. . . Well, I had asked, and they delivered."

Everyone knew Gary's name. The employees at the hotel always greeted Gary with, "Hi, Gary," not with "Hello, sir."

"Gary liked people knowing his name," Carol said.

It made him feel like himself.

"This was an exciting time for us," Carol said. "We had been waiting so long to tell everyone what they did to us."

Miller offered to have a driver pick up Gary every day, but some days the traffic at 8:30 in the morning was so bad their ride had trouble getting to the courthouse on time. The Freddie Gray trial—a case about the police-involved death of a black man—was attracting reporters, cameramen, and spectators from all over the world.

"It was faster to walk," Carol said. "It depended on how Gary was feeling."

Also, Gary didn't want to get into anyone's car, because he could have an accident, and he didn't want it to smell up their car.

"He would have accidents getting out of cars," Carol said. "And every time he would take a step, some body fluid would come out, and so I would put things down on the wheelchair. I would have extra with me so that I would be able to change him and clean everything up. And I also have deodorizer with me so that he wouldn't have to be embarrassed that anyone but me would smell it. He was more comfortable with me walking him, even though he hated it because he knew I had a suitcase, my purse, a throw up bucket, and I was wheeling him up a hill and then down a hill, and then back up a hill each time. And the bumps. I would have to stop if it got to be too painful for him, and he didn't want anyone else to notice that he was in a wheelchair. He wanted to be invisible."

Carol made sure Gary didn't see how hard it was to wheel him back and forth to the courthouse.

On really bad days, they didn't go to court.

# 92

The hotel was two blocks from Angelos's office, which it made it easy for Miller to stop by after court.

"My recollection [about the jury] is we had four African-American women, one white woman, and one white male, that was the six," Miller said.

Miller tried to read the jurors: which ones would be sympathetic to Gary's case.

"I got to be honest with you," Miller said, "the scary part for me was, I couldn't get anything from this jury."

He couldn't read them.

"They were paying attention," Miller said, "but I couldn't get a read on any of them." Carol kept saying, "This jury is with you." I said, "Maybe you're seeing more than I am, Carol, because I don't see it. I'm not getting a feel. Sometimes jurors will do that."

One day, when Miller told the court that Gary couldn't be in court, a juror in the back row mouthed, "OMG is he ok?"

Miller said, "Yes, he is okay."

"I knew then she loved Gary," Miller said, "and she became the juror I spoke directly to for the rest of the trial."

During the closing argument, Miller would direct his argument to her.

# 93

"By late in the evening of May 12, 2011, Carol Stern had seen enough," Warshaw said in his opening statement. "She had watched her husband agonize in pain for a few days, and so she finally picked up the phone, called 911, and an ambulance came and transported him to Sinai Hospital. He arrived there with a complaint of severe abdominal pain, what medical people call abdominal pain, but laypeople may think of as a stomachache, or bellyache. It specifically, and what you will hear, significantly, that pain was located in the left upper quadrant of the abdomen. If you think of a line down the middle and down across your belly in four quadrants, it's in the left upper quadrant, and you will see that in the medical records. And you will also see that he described the pain as being sharp in nature, and burning in nature, and that it hurt more when he would breathe, or take a breath. We know now that Mr. Stern was suffering from an ulcer, and specifically an ulcer in his duodenum, and that's a medical term; the duodenum is where the stomach first attaches to the small intestine. And so he was admitted to Sinai Hospital for four days, and during those four days he was seen two times by the defendant, Todd Heller, who had been called in as a specialist in gastrointestinal illness or disease. But Dr. Heller failed to diagnose that ulcer, or why Mr. Stern had this left upper quadrant pain. And so when he was discharged four days later on May 17th, his ulcer had been undiagnosed and untreated, and needless to say, he did not get better. And eight days later, on May 25, 2011, another ambulance was called, and this time Mr. Stern was transported to Northwest Hospital up on Liberty Road. And he was admitted to the hospital again, and during this admission, he was seen by Dr. Epstein on May 26th, Dr. Heller's partner, they work together in the same practice group. By now, you will also hear that Mr. Stern had developed something called guarding, and you will find out from the medical testimony in the case, what that means is that when the doctor goes to press on the abdomen to see if there is any pain, the muscles tense up to protect against the pain, and they call that guarding. And that was a progression of this ulcer that he had developed. And this time it was Dr. Epstein who failed to diagnose or treat Mr. Stern's ulcer. Thirty-three hours after Dr. Epstein saw Mr. Stern at Northwest Hospital, that ulcer perforated during the early morning hours of May 28th, gastric content to seep out into his abdomen, where it does not belong. He became very ill as a result, and he required surgery and suffered complications from that surgery that I will talk about in further detail, that required him to have approximately two dozen surgeries, surgical procedures over the next two years, including four bowel resections, meaning having parts of his small bowel and the large bowel removed. And by the way, the term bowel is synonymous with intestines, so small intestine is the same thing as small bowel, large intestine is the same thing as the large bowel. And for the large bowel, you may also hear that referred to as the colon. But he had four resections over those two years, and now he is left with a condition called short bowel syndrome. He does not have enough bowel to process food, and so he is on what's called TPN, and you will hear more about that during the trial, but it's essentially tube feeding, and that's how he gets all his nutrition. You will hear that he lives in chronic pain.

"He has a pain pump, he cannot walk without some manner of assistance, other than maybe very short distances. And he is totally dependent on others for his care and survival. This case is about the defendants' failure to diagnose Mr. Stern's ulcer, and to treat that ulcer, leading to these horrific consequences for both [him] and his wife. As you heard during jury selection, my name is Mike Warshaw, and along with my colleague, Jay Miller, we represent Gary and Carol Stern in this case."

Warshaw described Gary's childhood and career: A hometown kid, Towson State University, while he worked part time at Wendy's, the bar, the bail bonds company, which was—Warshaw said—located in the building next door, the Court Square building.

"Medically speaking," Warshaw said, "Gary was generally healthy, with one notable condition: he had been diagnosed with Crohn's Disease. I know you have heard that term in the jury selection process. He was diagnosed with Crohn's Disease in his early teens; that is a disorder that causes inflammation in the gastrointestinal tract, and mostly that occurs where what's called the terminal ileum, or the end of the small bowel . . . connects to the large bowel, or the colon, and this area is called the cecum. The bottom part of the small intestine is called the ileum, and so when you put the two together, it's called the ileocecal junction. And you will see, that's in the right lower quadrant, if you divide it. That's where Crohn's Disease typically occurs, and that's where Mr. Stern's Crohn's Disease was located. And you will hear from him when he testifies that growing up, as a result of this condition, he had to carefully watch his diet. He took medications for it over a number of years, and in the year 2000—he was thirty-seven years old at that time—he had that ileocecal junction removed. He had a surgery and it was taken out. And from that point in 2000, all the way to the time we get to the facts in this case, in 2011, Mr. Stern's Crohn's Disease was in complete remission."

He described how Gary and Carol met, how they married, their home in Owens Mills, and when Gary's pain started in early May 2011. He described Gary's nausea, vomiting, and diarrhea.

It was clear the jury would be spared no biological details no matter how embarrassing it might be for Gary. Carol knew the jury had to know the worst.

# 94

Warshaw described the ambulance trip to Sinai Hospital late on the evening of May 12, 2011, and what happened there, the first doctor's examination and his differential diagnosis.

"Doctors use that term," Warshaw explained. "Differential diagnosis is simply a list of potential diagnoses."

Differential diagnoses may include gastritis, which covers anything related to the stomach; reflux, which includes anything related to the esophagus; pancreatitis, which includes the pancreas; and peptic ulcer disease, which includes either a gastric ulcer in the stomach or a duodenal ulcer in the duodenum.

About 4:45 in the morning of May 13, Gary was admitted to the hospital.

Warshaw described Dr. Johnson-Futrell, who noted Gary's complaint of left upper quadrant pain—which would suggest an ulcer. And he told the jury how during Gary's time at Sinai, nobody did any tests on Gary for an ulcer, such as an endoscopy.

Warshaw talked about Drs. Heller and Epstein, the gastroenterologists from Woodholme Gastroenterology. He described Heller's first examination of Gary at 9:00 on the morning of May 14.

"You will hear that Dr. Heller would review the medical record, the chart that was already there," Warshaw said, "and he would see Dr. Peoples's note from the emergency room, Dr. Johnson-Futrell's note from the admission. He would take a history from Mr. Stern, asking him questions about what was going on, what's gone on in the past. He would perform his own physical examination and review diagnostic studies."

The only positive finding was tenderness in the left upper quadrant, which was apparently dismissed because it didn't fit in with the Crohn's diagnosis. The CAT scan indicated no inflammation in the colon, in the large or small bowel.

"In fact," Warshaw said, "the radiologist who issued that final [CAT scan report] stated, 'Findings do not suggest active disease.' Despite that, when Dr. Heller wrote to Dr. Johnson-Futrell, he indicated that Gary was suffering from Crohn's Disease."

On Gary's next visit, Dr. Heller did not order any testing of Gary's upper abdomen or left upper quadrant. He decided Gary was suffering a Crohn's flare, "despite," Warshaw said, "the absence of evidence of that."

Warshaw said that "It was a breach in standards of care by Dr. Heller to not even consider that this may have been peptic ulcer disease, or gastritis, or something else in the upper GI tract . . . Standard of care required that a proper and full evaluation of Mr. Stern required upper endoscopy."

All the GI experts who were going to testify—Warshaw said—"will all agree that if an upper endoscopy procedure had been performed during the hospitalization on May 13 to May 17, 2011, it would have revealed the presence of a duodenal ulcer. And if found" and treated "it would have healed, and that would have been the end of the story."

At the end of Warshaw's opening statement, he added, "I just want to alert you, as we have discussed with the Court and counsel, with no disrespect meant to anybody, there are times where Mr. Stern won't be here, because he can't."

# 95

Penhallegon, the lawyer for the defense, gave his opening argument.

"This is an important case," he said. "It's an important case for Mr. and Mrs. Stern, and I can promise you, it is an important case for Dr. Heller and for Dr. Epstein. You might remember, there was a movie that came out some years ago, for those of you who are younger than I, there was an actor by the name of Michael J. Fox, and he played a character by the name of Marty McFly, who through a time machine—it was a car called a DeLorean— with this time machine, he was able to go back in time and he ended up back at a time when his now parents were still in high school. And Marty's job was to make sure, having now gone back in time, that his parents met each other and dated and married, so that the future could turn out the way that Marty knew it was. And one of the reasons why these kinds of movies are entertainment for us, and are so popular, is because they are so different than the way real life is. In real life, none of us have that advantage of going back in time with the knowledge of what has happened in the future. And I submit to you that what you are going to find in this case is that this is a case where the plaintiff's medical witnesses are using the benefit and the wisdom of hindsight, after Mr. Stern had surgery, to blame two doctors who had nothing to do with those operations. Dr. Heller and Dr. Epstein are not surgeons. . . Dr. Heller and Dr. Epstein are not . . . the physicians who admitted Mr. Stern to Sinai Hospital, they are not the physicians who discharged him."

Penhallegon's defense was that Heller and Epstein were asked only to consult. They were not ultimately responsible for the mistakes that left Gary in the condition he was in.

Penhallegon's description of Gary's hospital history more or less matched Gary's and Carol's lawyer's timeline. The question wasn't what happened, but who was responsible.

"The question that you will ultimately need to decide," Penhallegon said, "is whether the recommendations that they made with the information they then had—not with back to the future hindsight—were reasonable, and the evidence is going to show not only were they reasonable, but they proved to be correct."

Penhallegon told the jury he would "have an opportunity to address you one final time," during his closing statement, "and I will at that point respectfully ask that you return your verdict in favor of Todd Heller, and in favor of Steve Epstein. Thank you very much."

## 96

At the hotel, Carol made sure Gary was comfortable and saw to his medication and clothing. When she came out of the shower, Gary was looking at the harbor.

"I must have been standing there watching him for five minutes or so," Carol said. "I knew I needed to move, but I couldn't help but think I was looking at the perfect man and the perfect picture. I was looking at a miracle. My husband was alive and at peace. I didn't ever want to forget. I picked up my phone and took a picture; then, I walked over to him and put my hand on his lower back. He turned his head to look at me."

"I love you," Carol said.

"I love you, too, Baby Doll," Gary said.

"What are you looking at?"

"Life."

"And it's good."

"Life is great with you in it."

"Life is great with us together."

"You know we're going to win this case."

"Yes, I know."

"I'm going to make sure you have everything you ever wanted."

"I already do, Babe," Carol said. "I have you, and you're alive, and you're going to stay that way."

"Whatever you say, Baby Doll," Gary said.

## 97

"After opening arguments, I was really amazed how both sides seemed to really do their homework," David said. "I kept looking at Judge Cannon, who my father, Sonny, appeared before, but I couldn't say anything as it may have been a conflict of interest."

David looked at the jurors, wondering how they were going to take all this in. Would they be able to understand all the twists and turns? The subtle distinctions involved?

"Would they make a rash decision?" David wondered. "I felt like it could go either way. During the trial, it seemed the other attorneys countered everything we were saying . . . I miss my brother."

During Miller's cross-examination of Dr. Johnson-Futrell, Miller asked, "When you saw Mr. Stern in May, you had been practicing just for a month?"

"I believe so," Dr. Johnson-Futrell said, "yes."

"Gary would have been the first, or one of the very few patients with a question of Crohn's Disease, or peptic ulcer disease, that you would have seen?" Miller asked.

Miller was establishing the kind of care Gary received at Sinai.

He questioned Dr. Johnson-Futrell about her shift, from 7:00 p.m. to 7:00 a.m.

"Through the night," Miller asked. "Right?"

"Yes."

"And your role as a hospitalist over the night . . . was to admit patients from the emergency department into the hospital, correct?"

"Yes."

"And in that role, you understood that when you admitted a patient like Mr. Stern, you were not going to follow him through his admission, correct?"

"Exactly, yes."

"Someone else . . . would pick up his care after you admitted him?"

"Yes."

Miller's case depended on trying to clarify where responsibility lay for what happened to Gary; the mistaken diagnosis of Crohn's and the absence of any treatment for Gary's ulcer.

And where it did not lie.

"You also requested a gastroenterology consult, correct?"

"Yes."

"And that's because there was this question about Crohn's Disease, which falls into the GI field of expertise, correct?"

"Yes."

What Miller was trying to prove was that from the moment Gary entered the emergency room, the default assumption seemed to be that Gary was suffering from Crohn's—which was not challenged. It became the consensus reality, passed by one caregiver to another like a street legend.

"And," Miller asked, "you're going to involve [a gastroenterologist] because you want their particular expertise for those types of illnesses?"

"Yes," Dr. Johnson-Futrell said.

Miller was putting up a signpost aiming at who was responsible.

"Now," Miller said, "when you did admit Mr. Stern with your evaluation, including this exacerbation of Crohn's Disease, you were, in part . . . relying upon the preliminary CT . . . "

"Yes."

"And that's preliminary because that was read by someone, I think they are referred to as nighthawks?"

"Yes, overnight radiologists." Who could be anywhere in the world. Through the internet, doctors in one hospital could reach out and get help from experts a continent away—which means the pool of expertise could be as wide as possible, but at the cost of loss of intimacy, of direct contact.

The analysis is sent to the off-site experts, who can—as Miller pointed out—give Dr. Johnson-Futrell "an early impression before the staff radiologist at Sinai comes back in the morning – "

"Yes."

" —and gives their full, final reading, right?"

The doctors at Sinai had fallen into the trap of assuming a diagnosis and then looking for evidence that the diagnosis was correct.

"Yes."

"And together, that's how [doctors] interpreted what you were seeing from the overnight read?"

"Yes."

"You did not have the final CT scan report, correct?" Miller asked.

"Not," Dr. Johnson-Futrell said, "not at that time."

"And so you were not aware that in the final read," Miller said, "there was no acute inflammatory changes noted, correct?"

"No," Dr. Johnson-Futrell said.

"And are you aware of the fact that in the course of this case," Miller asked, "Mr. Stern has denied stating that this episode had been similar to a prior flare?"

"No," Dr. Johnson-Futrell said. "I didn't know that."

"Now," Miller asked, "when you evaluated Mr. Stern, you mentioned the soft abdomen, I think that's where you told us that that helped rule out some of the things . . . specifically you mentioned a perforation . . ."

"Um hmm."

" . . . of an ulcer."

"Yeah."

" . . . ruled out a perforation," Miller said, "but it didn't rule out the possibility of an ulcer, did it?"

"No," Dr. Johnson-Futrell said, "I don't believe you can rule that out by exam only."

After Miller questioned Dr. Johnson-Futrell about the rest of her analysis of Gary's condition, he told the judge, "Your Honor, I have nothing further at this time."

"Any redirect?" the judge asked

"No redirect, Your Honor," Penhallegon said.

The witness was excused.

Gary and Carol knew the case had to be built, but they were frustrated that what was so obvious to them wasn't immediately clear: how Gary was not treated for what he suffered from and was treated for a condition he didn't have, which led to Gary's current condition.

# 98

There were days the trial seemed to go on and on.

"It was so tiring," Carol said, "Gary and I would go back to the hotel and order room service, then Gary would go to sleep, and I would just sit there, look out at the water until Gary would wake up and need something. But other days, we both would be so excited about court. Miller would always stop by or call us to see if we needed anything and to tell us about what was going to happen the next day."

David would often come down to the hotel after he got off work.

"We would sit around the deck on the second floor," Carol said, "and talk about how the trial was going. Gary would be so excited when Miller showed how the other side screwed up."

"See, see," Gary said to Miller. "I told you so, they gave me the wrong medication, then cut me open like a fish. They couldn't even bother doing an endoscopy on me, a ten-minute test, bunch of assholes, and now I'm like this."

"Gary," David said, "I know we're showing them now you were right all along."

"Ya," Gary said. "But look at me."

"Gary," Carol warned, "you're getting too excited."

"Look at what they did to *you*," Gary said.

Gary took the stand on August 20, 2015, at 9:27 a.m.

Miller asked Gary how often he used his wheelchair.

Gary said, "Pretty much all the time. It's very hard to get around. I have a lot of, as you can see, a lot of apparatuses I have to wear. I have to bring my feeding tube sixteen hours a day, and I have a pain pump that runs 24/7, so it's pretty hard to, with my strength, which isn't much these days, it's hard for me to like put on like a knapsack or something like that. And it, I really can't go very far."

"Now," Miller asked, "if it wasn't for all that apparatus, would you still have difficulty moving around a lot?"

"Absolutely," Gary said.

"And why?" Miller asked.

"Well, it's because I have no more stomach muscles, so right now my, basically my insides are on my outsides, just covered by a thin layer of skin. And the biggest fear is that if somebody even jerks, so I can't put a seatbelt on, a sudden stop, if it penetrates that it will kill me, it would just go right through [my skin] and my guts will be all over the place, unfortunately. And I don't mean to say it like that, but it's just the way it is, so it's very hard, it's very limited places I can go. I don't have the strength, I mean, I'm just so worn down from all these surgeries, and all this."

"I don't want to embarrass you this morning," Miller said, "so I'm not going to ask you to lift your shirt up, but I want you to describe to the jury, and we do have some photos later, but I'm going to do it when you're not here. Just tell them what your, when you say you have no stomach muscles, what does your belly look like?"

"I'm sorry, it's very humiliating. I look like I'm about six months pregnant."

"So it sticks out?"

"The best way to put it, it just, it's like I'm six months pregnant. It's very odd, it's in different shapes, different forms, very deformed. It sinks in, it sinks out, and you can literally watch something I eat. I ate like a piece of cookie and watch it go down whatever bowel I have left."

"You can see your bowel through the surface of your skin?"

"You can see the food moving through it, yes."

Miller asked Gary about his life: where he was born, where he went to school, the bar, the bail bonds business with David, his former case of Crohn's.

"Did you have any real problems in 2000 up until the time of this admission that we're here about in May of 2011?" Miller asked.

"No," Gary said, "not a thing. I was healthier than I've ever felt."

"We heard Mr. Warshaw talk about this lady sitting back here, Mrs. Stern, that's your wife?"

"That's my angel."

Gary described how they met, fell in love, married.

"And then I know you have some memory issues, so I'm going to help you, you got married in 2006?"

"I believe so, yes."

"So you've been married what, nine, ten years?"

"I can remember the date, May 1st. I get points for that, don't I?"

"Yes, you do. I take it from 2006 when you got married, to this admission in 2011, tell the jury about your marriage, was it good? Happy?"

"The best."

Gary described moving to North Carolina, who lived with him and Carol—and Butchy, who (Gary explained) "has learned how to sense me when I got sick . . . He must have learned my mannerisms as they got worse, because it's amazing how he will know like minutes before I have a seizure, and my wife might be sleeping, he will drag the blanket off of me, up to her, and scratch at her. *Somethings wrong, something's wrong*, to wake her up . . . I'm going to the bathroom a lot, which I am now these days, and if for some reason I have a seizure going to the bathroom, whatever, he knows to go there and get her and bring her."

Gary talked about going to the Sinai Emergency Room on May 13 and what happened there, how they seemed to not pay attention to his description of where the pain was, and how different it was from his Crohn's pain.

"Was this pain in your left upper quadrant similar to the pain you had in 2000?"

"Absolutely not . . . I thought I was having a heart attack. It wasn't anything with Crohn's, I never thought it was Crohn's . . . I was telling them, I said, 'This is not my Crohn's, I'm telling you right now. I feel like I'm more like having a heart attack.'"

Miller said, "We have a Dr. Simon coming in and a Dr. Nock who is going to go through your records in detail, but I want to pick out a few items. Do you recall the time in between surgeries when you had an ostomy, colostomy bag? Where your bowels were connected to a bag?"

"There are times, we . . ."

"You don't have a good recollection of it?"

Gary explained he was hazy about some specifics because "they had me under medications and stuff . . . "

"How long, if you recall, has it been that you had this short bowel where you cannot get any nutrients from any food that you eat?" Miller asked. "A year? Two years?"

"Probably closer to three years now," Gary said.

" . . . What kind of device do you have going into your body that gives you nutrition?"

"Well, I have a permanent, what's this called, a Hickman, which is a permanent IV right here, which is, they put it in one of my big veins right here, and I can have two to three ports come out where I can administrate my feeding bags, my IV medicines, and stuff like that, my pain medicines, stuff like that."

"Do you have a surgical tube that's in your artery permanently . . ."

"Correct."

" . . . stitched in there and then there's a hole available on the outside?"

"Correct, it's two like little IV things you would see if you went into the hospital and they put, they always put the saline bottle in the little thingy in your arm, it's sort of like that, but they're always hanging out, because it's sewn into my, one of my main arteries in my, 24/7."

"And is that device how you get your nutrition from what we've been calling TPN?"

"Correct, that's how basically I live. If I don't have that nutrition pumping inside of me, and it all has to be calibrated, every single week they have to take my blood to see whether my blood is, sugar's too high, I've never had diabetes in my life, and all of a sudden I'm having problems with diabetes because it's very sugar and protein oriented, and you know, it can send my sugar this way, that way. So if it wasn't for my wife, and from her learning on the job . . . I would be dead . . . "

"And how often is that TPN delivered to your home?"

"Every seven days. It's got to be tweaked every seven days, so they take blood out of me every seven days, cultures, whatever they need to do, and it's delivered every seven days, and two days out of the five, out of the seven days, every week, we sit around all day, waiting for the UPN guy to deliver my medications. It's part of our living now."

"In fact, you've had to make arrangements while you're here for delivery to the hotel and to get tested and adjusted, and those sort of things, haven't you?"

"Absolutely. Had to set all that up before we left . . . I have to go to LabCorp to get some blood done . . . And they have to send the medications, all my food, and my bags and everything, to the hotel where we're staying."

"How long is that TPN giving you medication in a twenty-four-hour period?"

"It's on sixteen hours a day."

"Now, in addition to the TPN, you mentioned a pain pump. Does that go in at the same line, but a different port?"

"Exactly, yes."

"Sort of like having an electrical outlet with two sockets?"

"Exactly, yes."

"And how often is your pain pump operating?"

"It's . . . a very, very slow trickle . . . It's on almost twenty-four hours a day, sometimes [Carol] will turn it off when I go to sleep . . . if the pain is not killing me. . . Just enough to knock that edge off. But it's still there, everybody tells me it will never go away anymore, so I don't know what that means anymore."

"Now, Mr. Warshaw described in the opening that you eat for pleasure, because you don't get any nutrients from it, but I don't get the idea it's very pleasurable. . . Tell us what your eating is like. Have you eaten a porterhouse steak recently?"

Gary laughed and said, "No . . . I used to love steamed crabs, stuff like that, all good Baltimore cooked stuff. I used to weigh a hundred and forty-five pounds, and I'm down to like a hundred and five pounds." The eating "is purely for pleasure. . . It's just like one or two bites, just for that taste . . . If I swallow it, I'm taking a chance."

"What happens if you eat a steak?"

"It's got to be more like a pureed kind of thing, like put it in a blender, you puree it, you know? . . . I can't eat no seeds, or nothing like that, nothing that will catch whatever little bit of bowel I have left, because that can cause all kinds of problems if it gets caught."

"Now," Miller said, "forgive me, but you have some issues with your bowels."

Gary said, "Um hmm."

"Can you tell us about that?"

"As far as . . . ?"

"Well . . ."

". . . now?"

". . . you spend a lot of time in the bathroom. Do you find yourself having to move your bowels a lot, even with the TPN and not eating a lot . . . ?"

Carol knew how embarrassing it was for Gary to discuss publically such private matters. But Gary didn't hesitate or use euphemisms.

"I have forty-two centimeters left of my bowel," he said. "I have half of my colon left. It doesn't hold much . . . Everything I eat and drink by mouth just goes *phhhsstt*, right through, like a river."

"And you have issues controlling it as well," Miller asked, "do you not?"

Carol winced.

"Especially at night time," Gary said. "It's very humiliating. I have a lot of accidents at nighttime . . . Just, it's just, I don't know, it's just very humiliating to, you know, you wake up and you're in a pile of, you know, you're in feces, or you're in stuff like that again, and you're just thinking to yourself . . . why is this happening, why is this happening to me? What did I do to deserve this?"

"Why can't you wear adult diapers, like Depends?"

"Again, it goes back to earlier, I can't wear zipper pants, I can't wear buckle pants, I can't wear a seatbelt, it's because I have about two inches of skin and that's it, covering my belt here now."

"So even something that is a diaper doesn't work?"

"It's going to push it, it pressures it in, it pushes in, which gives me massive pain."

"So you . . . can't even stand the pain from a diaper?"

"No."

"Same thing with maybe. . ."

"Any kind of pressure."

"You don't wear underwear? You can't wear anything . . ."

"No underwear, absolutely not."

"So therefore, you are prevented from wearing the diapers that would give you some less embarrassment."

"With the accidents at least."

Carol thought Gary's candor revealed how gallant he was.

"You mentioned to me that that's why you're . . . not eating at all while this trial is going on, right?"

"Trying not to."

"I apologize for . . . I want to know, can you, do you need help in the morning when you get up? Do you need help dressing yourself?"

"I do."

"Why?"

"That's my weakest part of the day . . . If I get a lot of sleep, which is not very often, my wife is . . . the biggest angel in the world . . . She's staying up all night . . . taking care of me, or administrating medicines every six or twelve hours, this, that, and the other, and she lived in the hospital with me for three and a half years. Straight. Didn't leave one day, that's how long I was in the hospital for that one stretch. My stomach was wide open. She did not leave. She . . . bought a bed at Wal-Mart and put it next to me, and she learned on-the-job . . . training from all the nurses and the doctors how to do all this so she could take me home and take care of me . . . But, it's just too much. She's killing herself doing this . . . It's . . . not fair to her . . ."

Gary continuously emphasized not *his* distress but Carol's.

"When you use the restroom, are you able to do that by yourself?"

"Getting to it is probably the worst part. Once I'm sitting, once you're sitting, get settled on it, I can usually go."

But, Gary explained, he had trouble reaching around to clean himself, "so she does help me with that, too."

"It sounds like your wife is with you 24/7, that there's not really much she can do right now outside the home and leave you?"

"Twenty-four/seven, she is there. She's been to the hospital six times herself because of this, because of exhaustion. Taking care of me! And I'm just afraid that something is going to happen, it's just not fair. She didn't sign up for this, I didn't sign up for this."

## 99

"Gary," Miller asked, "how has this affected your feelings as a husband?"

"My husband was the most loving, and caring, and thoughtful man I had ever met in my entire life," Carol, outside court, would later say," and all he did was love me. No matter what, he loved me. And he would just show it in the most simple ways. We didn't have to have massive sex all the time, although it was good . . . We had crazy sex outside my apartment, underneath the light on his black Corvette, in the middle of the night, and after we were done we heard applause, so we bowed and went up to my apartment. But it wasn't about that with us, it was about the fact that he could start a sentence and I could finish it, because I knew what he was thinking, because we were, we were one person. I didn't have to see or feel the physical pain that he was feeling, I felt it in my heart, he felt it in his entire body."

After Gary got sick, especially when his internal organs were exposed, they would talk about sex the way they would talk about food: what they would do when Gary got well.

"We got frisky," Carol would say.

"Not much, not much at all," Gary, in court, answered Miller's question about how his disease affected his feelings as a husband.

"I don't know why she, sometimes I just don't know why she's still here, why she would want to go through all this. But, like I said, she's my angel. Somebody sent her here to do this for me, I guess. I don't know how else to explain it. I would be dead if it wasn't for her. She's [brought] me back three times from coding, at my home."

Wisely, Penhallegon told the judge he had no questions. There was nothing he could ask that would not make him unsympathetic.

"It was very difficult to have to watch my brother and best friend live every second of the past five years with people torturing him," David said after Gary testified. "And he has to wonder if the jury was going to believe what we are saying all the while the other side—the lawyers—were making this whole thing up, making it seem like this whole ordeal was no big deal, and that someone else caused all this. They tried to minimize everything, and all Gary could do is put his head down and shake his head. He would never let someone take advantage of him or someone in his family. I'll say it again, we knew the truth all along. We just needed to prove it."

# 100

After the recess, Warshaw called Dr. Todd Heller to the stand. He ran through Dr. Heller's background and then asked about his examination of Gary.

"I mentioned in the opening to the jury, something called endoscopy," Warshaw said. "Can you explain what endoscopy is?"

"Endoscopy is a general term referring to placing a tube into an orifice," Heller said.

"And specifically for a gastroenterologist such as yourself," Warshaw said, "endoscopy would include both colonoscopy and EGD, or upper endoscopy, correct?"

Warshaw was laying the ground for questioning why Heller did not check for an ulcer.

"You did not order an upper endoscopy, did you?" Warshaw said.

"That certainly would not be indicated at that point," Heller said.

Warshaw asked a few more questions about Gary's symptoms and how they fit or did not fit a Crohn's flare. Then:

" . . . when you saw Mr. Stern on this visit," Warshaw asked, "you still have no diagnostic study to indicate that he was having an acute flare of Crohn's, did you?"

"No," Dr. Heller said, "that's why we wanted to eventually colonoscope him."

"Gary <u>was,</u> however, complaining about 'persistent left upper quadrant pain' and still, even seeing him again with these studies returned, you did not order a study of his upper gastrointestinal tract, did you?"

"No," Dr. Heller said, "I didn't."

There was more back and forth, during which Dr. Heller struck Carol as stonewalling.

But Warshaw went in for the kill: "Can we agree now, Dr. Heller, that when you saw Mr. Stern on May 13, 2011 and May 14, 2011, that he did in fact have a duodenal ulcer?"

"I don't know that he did or not," Dr. Heller said.

Carol wanted to scream.

"You do not?" Warshaw acted incredulous.

"I," Dr. Heller said, "I don't know."

A second time Dr. Heller seemed to hesitate: "I, I don't know." A <u>tell,</u> Carol thought: Dr. Heller knew he wasn't being candid.

"You certainly didn't diagnose it," Warshaw said, "did you?"

"No," Dr. Heller said.

"Nothing further," Warshaw said.

Carol figured Dr. Heller had indicted himself. Would the jury think so?

# 101

During cross-examination, Penhallegon asked questions about Dr. Heller's background, focusing on his expertise in his field.

Penhallegon asked Dr. Heller to define Crohn's Disease.

"Crohn's Disease is an inflammatory condition of the digestive system," Dr. Heller answered. "It can occur anywhere from mouth to rear end. But why it occurs, bottom line, we don't know."

"People don't know what causes it?" Penhallegon asked.

"There may be genetic influences, or whether they were environmental or dietary influences is not really well established, and to treat it, but the bottom line, we don't have a great knowledge as to what causes it."

"And so let me ask you this and repeat the words rightly if I can. Does a complaint of pain or tenderness in the left upper quadrant suggest a duodenal ulcer?"

"No," Dr. Heller said.

"Why not?"

"It's not in the typical region where one would have pain from a duodenal ulcer."

*This*—Carol thought—*is a misdirection and a circular argument.* Dr. Heller seemed to be saying that an ulcer would not present in the area he chose to examine (an area that might suggest Crohn's), not in the area he did not choose to examine (the area where Gary said he was experiencing pain).

Dr. Heller described the colon as looking "like a question mark."

*Perfect,* Carol thought. *A question mark. That's what the trial was about. Answering the question, what happened inside Gary.*

# 102

On most breaks in the trial, Carol took Gary downstairs and out of the building so Gary could get some sun and Carol could grab a smoke. Outside, they saw members of the jury. But they kept at a distance.

On one of the first few days, their lawyer Miller came over to them and asked, "Gary, are you smoking?"

"Why would you ask that?" Gary said.

"The other side will make a big deal about that," Miller said.

Carol knew an assistant attorney from the other side was behind her.

"Let them," Carol said. The assistant attorney went back into the courthouse.

"I think he was listening to us," Miller said.

"I know he was," Carol said.

She gestured down the block where half the jury members were smoking.

"You're bad," Miller said.

"No," Carol said. "I'm mad."

"Don't mess with her," Gary said.

"I knew that," Miller said. "But now I see it firsthand."

# 103

After lunch, Warshaw called the other defendant, Dr. Steven Epstein.

"Good afternoon, Dr. Epstein," Warshaw said after Dr. Epstein was sworn in. ". . . [Y]ou mentioned you are a gastroenterologist, and like Dr. Heller, your employer is Woodholme Gastroenterology in Pikesville, correct?"

"Yes," Dr. Epstein said.

"And fair to say," Warshaw said, "again like Dr. Heller, you have no recollection of Mr. Stern as your patient?"

"Correct," Dr. Epstein said.

"So whatever we talk about would be what comes from the medical record itself?"

"Correct, I only saw him that one day, yeah."

After going through material about his examination of Gary, Warshaw asked Dr. Epstein, "And you would agree with Dr. Heller, I take it, that you would not limit your examination of Mr. Stern to just whether or not he had Crohn's Disease, you would do a full GI evaluation?"

"Absolutely," Dr. Epstein said. "Right, absolutely."

Warshaw pointed out that since Gary's surgery in 2000 he "had been doing quite well, had not been on any Crohn's-specific medications?"

"Yes," Dr. Epstein said.

"Burning pain like [Gary's] describing here," Warshaw said, "and sharp pain that he described from Sinai is more consistent with ulcer disease, is it not?"

The CT scan indicated "no evidence of colonic or small bowel inflammation to suggest an active Crohn's flare, right?" Warshaw asked.

"Correct," Dr. Epstein said, "based on the CT, correct."

*Passing the buck,* Carol thought. *What is wrong with these guys? They're holding someone's life in their hands, and yet they take no responsibility.*

"And your conclusion with reading that report," Warshaw asked, "was that that CT scan did not show any acute inflammatory changes, right?"

"Yeah," Dr. Epstein said.

"But," Warshaw said, "you had no evidence at that point, no objective evidence at that point to suggest that he was having a Crohn's flare, did you?"

Dr. Epstein talked around the question, leading up to him explaining "the day after [he saw Gary] was not my day to be there, so I wasn't involved, you know, after those days, after that day."

Nothing to see. Move along. Just a bystander.

"You also did not order any testing or studies, what have you, of Mr. Stern's upper gastrointestinal tract?" Warshaw asked.

"Correct," Dr. Epstein said.

"Specifically you did not order upper endoscopy?"

"Correct."

"You, in fact, did not even consider that he might have an ulcer," Warshaw asked, "did you?"

"Not at that time," Dr. Epstein said.

# 104

"Dr. Epstein," Penhallegon said in his cross-examination, "you mentioned that the treatment for peptic ulcer disease is a PPI, a proton pump inhibitor, is that right?"

"Correct," Dr. Epstein said.

PPI are drugs that reduce stomach acid.

"Is Protonix one of the types of PPI's?"

"Yes."

Penhallegon showed Dr. Epstein one of the exhibits.

"Now, do you recognize this as being a page from the Northwest Hospital Center medical records for this admission?"

"Yes."

"And does this page include medication orders that have been entered by the attending physicians and others?"

"Yes."

"The second order on this list is an order for Protonix . . ."

"Yes."

". . . that proton pump inhibitor? And according to this note, that order was first entered on what date and time?"

"May 26, 2011 at 5:02 a.m."

"Now, this is about ten hours or so, ten or eleven hours before you did your consult?"

"Yes."

Penhallegon was trying to establish that Dr. Epstein was not ultimately responsible for Gary's misdiagnosis.

Penhallegon questioned Dr. Epstein about Gary's condition: his C. difficile, his intussusception (which is when the small bowel collapses upon itself).

"It's sort of an accordion or telescoping is a good word," Dr. Epstein said.

Penhallegon asked Dr. Epstein, "You explained to Mr. Warshaw that this afternoon of May 26th, you did not order an upper endoscopy and didn't consider a peptic ulcer at that time?"

"Correct."

Penhallegon asked "How did Mr. Stern appear?"

"Yes," Dr. Epstein said, "I wrote, or I dictated, in general, the patient is walking around the room, appearing comfortable, in no acute distress."

In the redirect, Warshaw asked Dr. Epstein, "if you look through this medication administration record, you will agree with me that [Gary] had not received any proton pump inhibitor by the time you saw him at 3:30 on the 26th?"

"Correct," Dr. Epstein said, "because they just ordered it, right. I mean, it had just only been ordered."

"And when they went to fill the order, which should have been given before you got there, it wasn't available?"

"Correct."

". . . So when you said earlier that he was already started on Protonix, that wasn't actually true, because it hadn't been started yet, had it?"

"I guess at the time I saw that it was ordered, so."

"And again, you didn't mention that in your note to any extent, because peptic ulcer disease frankly wasn't a concern of yours as it pertained to this patient?"

"At that time it was not a topic. A diagnosis."

"But the fact of the matter is he had an ulcer, didn't he?"

"Based on what we know now, he did."

"It perforated about thirty-three, thirty-four hours after you saw him, right?"

"Um hmm," Dr. Epstein agreed.

"And based on that, we're pretty certain that it was there when you saw him, right?"

"Probably."

"And you didn't diagnose that, did you?"

"That wasn't on my list of diagnosis at the time."

*More evasion and buck passing,* Carol thought.

"That's all I have," Warshaw said.

Dr. Epstein was excused.

# 105

Gary was happy with what happened at the trial. He and Carol and David talked for an hour or so.

"Instead of going back to the room," Carol said, "we would all go over to the Inner Harbor and get some dinner at the Cheesecake Factory, with at least four slices of cheesecake for Gary to eat later that night. And, yes, Gary always paid for it later by spending half the night in the bathroom."

Gary would say "in a strong voice," according to Carol, "Things are going our way. It's our lucky day. Let's go over to the casino and play Black Jack."

"I don't think that's a good idea, Babe," Carol said.

"Why not? We can't lose today. Let's go."

Gary's willingness to risk going out on the town despite the possibilities of his having an accident proved to Carol Gary's hopeful mood. But Carol didn't think going to a casino was a good idea.

"I'm sorry but no," Carol said. "You get too excited, and you're liable to have a seizure."

"No," Gary said. "I'm not going to have a seizure."

"Yes," Carol said, "I know you're not because we're not going."

"Yes, we are."

"Okay, Gary, and what happens when you do, and you're back in the hospital instead of the court room? Do we really want to have the trial start all over?"

"No, Baby Doll."

"All right then. After we win—and we are going to win—we can go."

# 106

Miller called Dr. Bonnie Nock—who would testify about the recommendations she made for Gary's life care and needs, which would establish how much money it would cost, which in turn would affect a judgment on how much the court might award Gary if he won the case.

Miller went through Dr. Nock's background: a Bachelor of Science from the University of Pittsburgh and her studies at the North Texas State University for a Master's in physiology, which she finished while in medical school in 1988, when she got her doctorate in osteopathy. She was a resident in Internal Medicine at the Cleveland Clinic from 1989 to 1992, after which she spent three years as a resident at the Metro Health Medical Center in physical medicine and rehabilitation.

In coming up with a life plan for Gary, she worked with Evelyn Roberts, who, Dr. Nock, explained "has multiple roles. She is a case manager down in our area, and one of her other jobs is life care plans."

"Do you have an opinion to a reasonable degree of medical probability whether or not someone like Mr. Stern, or not Mr. Stern specifically, would do better at home or in an institution?" Miller asked.

Dr. Nock thought everyone does better at home than in an institution.

During cross-examination, Penhallegon asked, if "assistance in bathroom needs or self-grooming [was] an activity of daily living?"

"Yes," Dr. Nock said.

"Dressing in the morning, undressing in the evening, help with bed linens, and the like is an activity of daily living?"

"Yes."

"And those kinds of things, those kinds of daily assistance to Mr. Stern does not require a licensed nurse, does it?"

"No."

Penhallegon was suggesting that Gary would not need as much money as Miller would be asking for since he could make do with less intensive care.

" . . . a certified nursing assistant is perfectly able to provide assistance to Mr. Stern with regard to these activities of daily living, do you agree?"

"Yes."

"And you met, in addition to Mr. Stern, you met Mrs. Stern, am I right?"

"Yes."

"And she is currently providing much of the assistance with activities of daily living, am I right?"

"Yes."

"And she's doing an excellent job, agreed?"

"Yes."

Gary was incensed at the suggestion Carol would not need help.

"Do you have, based on your meeting with these folks, do you believe that Mrs. Stern wants to continue in assisting with her husband's care?"

"I think she feels she has to."

"Right, but even if there was a certified nursing assistant, an aide to provide respite so Mrs. Stern can go out and shop, or go to the salon, whatever she wants to do, do you think that Mrs. Stern wants to continue to be an active participant in her husband's care?"

"Yes."

Dr. Nock was excused.

# 107

The key argument was about whether or not Gary would need a full-time registered nurse, which would cost over $20 an hour. The defense claimed a licensed practical nurse—at $12 an hour—was good enough.

Miller was explaining that an LPN can't have anything to do with his pumps or medication or Gary's central line.

Privately, Miller asked Carol if an LPN could be sufficient to take care of Gary.

"Yes and no," Carol said. "Once I have everything done, Gary could go five hours without needing someone" to handle what an LPN could not do, if there were no problems. But, Carol added, there were always problems. For example, "Something goes wrong with the pumps all the time. An LPN can't touch it."

That night Gary and Carol talked about why they needed a registered nurse.

When something went wrong with the pump, an alarm would sound. A loud alarm.

"What if [the pump alarm] goes off in the court room," Gary said.

"We know how loud it is," Carol said.

"Ya," Gary said, "and so will they."

"Okay," Carol said, "so when . . ."

"When I hear them talking about only a LPN," Gary said, "I will clamp the line. The alarm will go off."

"Then," Carol said, "I will take you out of the courtroom." Gary was always cold, so Carol usually kept a blanket over his lap.

But the blanket would interfere with their demonstration.

The next day, when the question of a RN versus an LPN was raised, Gary clamped one of the tubes going into his body. The alarm shocked everyone in the court room.

Miller turned around and asked if Gary was okay.

"Yes," Carol said. "It's just one of his pumps."

# 108

---

Miller next called Evelyn Robert, a registered nurse, who had helped Dr. Nock develop a lifetime care plan for Gary, to the stand.

" . . . what is a life care planner?" Miller asked.

"A life care planner is a professional who determines through collaboration and assessment, and medical record review, and patient assessment, needs that are associated generally with either catastrophic or chronic illness, and you do that over a patient's lifetime," Ms. Roberts said. "You look at all their needs, you look at their medical, nonmedical" needs "associated with that specific diagnosis and sequalae from that diagnosis."

"And what is generally the purpose of that plan?" Miller asked.

"It's generally used in litigation, for the purpose of settlement."

"Do you agree with Dr. Nock that Mrs. Stern is doing a good job taking care of Mr. Stern?"

"She's doing an excellent job."

Miller asked if Carol was "able, in your opinion, physically to continue to be his sole caretaker 24/7?"

"When I met with Mrs. Stern, she was exhausted, distraught, overwhelmed, tearful many, many times. . . She wasn't sleeping."

Later on, in discussing the cost of services, Miller repeated his argument that Gary "may not have Medicare in the future. There was an argument made by counsel that we all are required to have insurance by the Affordable Care Act, that's the exact collateral source rule being argued. Why? Because if Donald Trump gets elected, he's going to repeal that act and we will no longer have a requirement, if we all . . ."

"Shhh," the judge said—although later she would respond to Miller's concern by suggesting that ". . . if by some miracle Donald Trump get[s] elected," she doubted he would get rid of Medicare.

# 109

The next day, Miller told the judge, "Mr. Stern is having some serious bowel issues . . . [Gary and Carol] are doing their best to get here. I would ask that you just tell the jury not details, [just] that he's having some medical issues and will be here when he can. I just don't want to leave them with the impression that they decided not to show up this morning."

The next witness Warshaw called was Dr. Todd Eisner, a gastroenterologist who did his undergrad studies at Brandeis University, went to medical school at the State University of New York at Stony Brook, did his internship and residency at North Shore University Hospital, Cornell Medical Center, and Sloan Kettering Cancer Center, where he also got a gastroenterology fellowship.

Warshaw asked Dr. Eisner to describe peptic ulcers, which, he explained, are ulcers of the upper gastrointestinal tract.

"The signs and symptoms would be abdominal pain, sometimes nausea, sometimes vomiting," Dr. Eisner said. "Sometimes the patient can have gastrointestinal bleeding as well. Typically the pain can be either after you eat, or a few hours after you eat."

The court accepted Dr. Eisner as an expert witness.

After going through Gary's condition, Warshaw asked, "Did Dr. Heller in his workup of Mr. Stern consider peptic ulcer disease as a potential diagnosis?"

"No," Dr. Eisner said.

"And do you have an opinion to a reasonable degree of medical certainty whether Dr. Heller breached standards of care applicable to him by failing to consider peptic ulcer disease in his differential diagnosis?"

"Yes," Dr. Eisner said, "he did."

"Do you have an opinion," Warshaw asked, "whether Dr. Heller breached applicable standards of care by failing to order any testing to explain the left upper quadrant pain?"

"Yes, I do," Dr. Eisner said. "The left upper quadrant pain . . . would not be explained by the diseases that he was being treated for, and he continued to have pain requiring narcotics, so what you want to do in that situation is evaluate the left upper quadrant pain, looking for an ulcer, whether it be like an ulcer in the stomach or of the small intestine."

"And in your opinion, Doctor, to a reasonable degree of medical certainty, what did standards of care require Dr. Heller to do in his care and treatment of Mr. Stern?" Warshaw asked.

"To order an endoscopy to evaluate the left upper quadrant pain," Dr. Eisner said.

"Do you have an opinion, Dr. Eisner, to a reasonable degree of medical certainty, if an upper endoscopy had been performed on Mr. Stern during this hospital admission, what it would have revealed?" Warshaw asked.

"I believe it would have revealed the duodenal ulcer that ultimately perforated a couple of weeks later," Dr. Eisner said.

After a break, Dr. Eisner said that, "If the duodenal ulcer would have been diagnosed and treated before it perforated, he would not have required surgery . . ."

During Dr. Eisner's cross-examination, Penhallegon asked, ". . . when you were first contacted and asked to look at this case, you had the benefit of knowing the outcome, true?"

"Yes," Dr. Eisner said.

"You had the benefit of, I think in medicine there's a principle called hindsight bias, have you heard of that?"

"Yes."

"And when one looks at whether the care provided by Dr. Heller was reasonable on May 14 and 15, would you agree that it would be unfair to judge his actions with any of the subsequent events?" Penhallegon asked.

"Yes," Dr. Eisner said, "certainly."

"Now, I think that you agree that there was a dramatic change in Mr. Stern's condition after these two doctors had last seen him, would you agree?"

"Yes, the dramatic change was the morning of the 28th."

" . . . And I think it's your opinion that the very early morning of May 28th, midnight, 12:30 in the morning or thereabouts, you believe that his duodenal ulcer perforated?

"Yes."

"And you've read [the surgeon's]operative reports?"

"Yes."

"[The surgeon] took Mr. Stern to the operating room on May 28th, right?"

"Yes."

"He did not find this perforation that you believe occurred some hours earlier, right?"

"Yes."

"And as a result of not finding it, he couldn't fix it, self-evident?"

"Correct."

"As a gastroenterologist, you have seen cases of perforated duodenal ulcers in the past, I assume?"

"Yes."

"They can be repaired, true?"

"Yes."

"Have you ever seen a patient with a perforated duodenal ulcer end up as a result of that having short bowel syndrome?"

"Not of the perforated duodenal ulcer in and of itself, no."

"Right. But in addition to not finding this ulcer, there was a second part of the operation that [the surgeon] did on May 28th, right?"

"Yes."

"And the second part of the operation was he resected, or cut out, a portion of Mr. Stern's small bowel and colon, right?"

"Yes."

"That portion of the operation had nothing to do with a duodenal ulcer, did it?"

"No."

"Did either of these two doctors from any of the records that you have seen ever suggest or recommend that a surgeon treat a possible Crohn's flare by going in and resecting and cutting out some of his bowel?"

"No."

"And I think what you said, I wrote it down. 'He didn't need surgery for Crohn's Disease.' Right?"

"Yes."

". . . Is it also your opinion, Dr. Eisner, that if [the surgeon] had never done that resection, that cut out of the bowel and colon, that we likely wouldn't be here today?" Warshaw said.

"I would say yes," Dr. Eisner said.

Penhallegon cross-examined Dr. Eisner.

". . . Crohn's Disease," Penhallegon said, "it never goes away, right?"

"Yes," Dr. Eisner said.

"And he then also says, 'This, meaning the patient's current episode, could represent a flare of the patient's Crohn's Disease,'" Penhallegon said, "and you agree it certainly could."

"Yes," Dr. Eisner said.

Penhallegon was establishing reasonable doubt for the jury. Maybe the defendants had not been negligent in Gary's treatment.

Carol thought it was a strong cross-examination.

# 110

Other witnesses testified about insurance, inflation, medicine, and money. At one point the judge thought Miller was getting too passionate about the case and once again told him, "Wait, take a chill pill, Mr. Miller. Mr. Miller, chill pill."

"What's . . .?" Miller started.

"Chill pill," the judge said.

"I'm chill," Miller said.

"Okay," the judge said. "And you see, you know when your partner is kicking you, it's chill pill time. Respond to your partner's kick."

"I'll start listening to my partner," Miller said.

"Okay," the judge said, "yes."

The question of the future of Medicare came up again.

". . . To tell you the truth," the judge said, "there would be no doubt in my mind that Medicare is going to be around. I mean, nobody's going to get rid of Medicare. I mean, if the country goes bankrupt, then you're going to get Medicare . . ."

They discussed Gary's life expectancy, which the judge said was "problematic . . . for me as a judge to decide, and I have some information about his life expectancy and I don't, I mean, if you're assessing him to say his life expectancy is ten years, I think it seems to me that would be, or five years, or whatever . . ."

A chilling discussion for Gary and Carol.

At one point, Miller apologized "for being testy."

"That's okay," the judge assured him, "no, no, no, you don't have to apologize to me."

Another witness—Dr. Thomas Borzilleri, a soft-spoken University of Maryland graduate, who was an economic consultant and economist— estimated how much Gary would need in future medical goods and services ("approximately $3.9 million)," general goods and services like "TPN and IV supplies, the power wheelchair and the van" (about $10.5 million), and "skilled nursing twenty-four hours a day" (about $405,150 per year).

He did not offer an opinion on how long Gary might live, which was a relief to Carol. She didn't want Gary to hear a low number and give up hope.

On the cross-examination, Penhallegon tried to establish a lower figure for Gary's future needs: If Gary lived for five more years, Penhallegon estimated Gary's expenses would be $5.9 million dollars (based in part on Evelyn Robert's life plan).

For Carol, this was worse than predictions of when Gary might die. They were trying to put a dollar value on Gary's life.

*Horrible*, she thought.

# 111

"It was the second week into the trial," Carol said. "Gary had a really bad night, and there was no way I was going to let him go to court."

Gary wanted to go. He did not want Carol to go alone. Carol called David and asked him to stay at the hotel with Gary while she went to the courtroom.

"David came running," Carol said, "just like he always did" when he was needed. "I couldn't stay away from Gary all day, so I waited until the afternoon session to show up in court.

"I had mixed emotions about being in court without Gary," Carol said. "However, he was feeling better. Gary always seemed to perk up anytime David was there. I think it was since they had moved to North Carolina, he didn't see David every day."

In the courtroom, Carol sat where she always sat, but without Gary's wheelchair next to her.

"I knew Gary was in good hands," Carol said, "but David has never been alone with Gary during a seizure."

Fortunately, Gary didn't have one.

"My body was in court," Carol said, "but my mind was on Gary. I couldn't even tell you who was on the stand."

About 2:30, Carol's phone started ringing.

"I know you're not supposed to have your phone on in a court room," Carol said, "and I didn't mean to have it on."

She had forgotten to turn it off or at least put it on vibrate.

"When I heard it ringing," Carol said, "so did everyone else. I know this because everyone except Jay looked at me."

Carol grabbed her purse and walked out of the courtroom "very fast."

"It was my sister Kendra wanting to know how things were going," Carol said.

After fifteen minutes, Carol went back into the court room. After court was let out for the day, she went up to the judge's clerk and said, "Could you please tell the judge I'm very sorry about not having my phone turned off. I respect her court room and didn't mean any disrespect."

The clerk said she would.

"The next day I had forgotten all about it," Carol said. "Gary was feeling better so we went to court together."

Gary, Carol, and Miller were in the courtroom before court started. The clerk walked over to Carol and said she had passed on Carol's apology about the phone call the day before, and the judge had said not to worry about it, she completely understood.

"Wow," Miller said, "Now, I've seen everything. This judge hates cell phones in her court. She's known for fining people for contempt and putting them in jail for getting phone calls in her court room."

"Well," Carol said, "it's off today."

# 112

When Carol was on the stand, Miller apologized for asking how old she was.

"Fifty-four," Carol said.

Miller ran through her background before and with Gary, including how her father went missing when she was young.

Miller asked her about her first marriage, about her children, Kenny and Kimberly, about Boston Market, and the Cantina—and about how they got their signals crossed, about how Gary didn't show up (because he was waiting at a different hot dog stand), how she waited until three o'clock in the morning.

"You obviously forgave him?" Miller said.

"Sometimes," Carol said. "We bring it up a lot. Sometimes."

Miller asked about why they moved to North Carolina.

"I needed help with Gary," Carol said, "and my son was willing to move in with us, and we had been in the Outer Banks before and the doctors told me that [Gary's] emotional status has a lot to do with him getting better, and it's calm down there and there's nothing out there, you can see all the stars."

Miller asked her about her grandchildren, Jade and Nadilla.

And he went through Gary's illness up to his admission in April of 2013 and since then.

Carol explained Gary had suffered many hospital admissions.

"For what?" Miller asked.

"Well," Carol said, "there's different reasons. If he gets an infection, then I take him into the emergency room, they evaluate him and they do cultures. If he's running a temperature, they will put him in the hospital for a couple of days, start the antibiotics until we can get him transferred home. He has been in the hospital for insulin seizures, benzo seizures, dehydration, different reasons. Not long stays, I think the longest stay has been like five or six days, and then I get him home as soon as possible."

"Who takes care of Gary on a daily basis?" Miller asked.

"I do," Carol said.

"How much help is Kenny able to give?"

"He gives me about an hour or two break so that I can take a shower, but I have to stay close by. He can watch Gary but if anything goes on with the pumps, I have to be right there to fix it because the pumps make him too nervous, there's too many things that could go wrong."

"I would like you to tell the jury about a typical day, a twenty-four-hour period when you wake up in the morning, I want you to take us through your day with Gary."

"It . . . starts at different times. I will wake up and Gary is screaming my name. If Gary has been asleep for more than a couple of hours he has accidents and he wakes up, and he needs me to get him to the bathroom and clean him up."

"I don't mean to, okay . . . "

"And I get him to the bathroom, I take his clothes, I put his sheets and everything in the washing machine, let the dogs out real fast, go back to Gary, see if he's okay. I check his sugar to see how his sugar has been, if I'm going to sleep for more than four hours, he needs his sugar checked every four hours . . ."

"I'm sorry."

"I ask him if he wants something to eat, he generally says no right away."

"Let me stop you. I want to try to learn what he can do for himself and what he can't. Is he able to, if you would hand him a washrag, can he clean himself up?"

"Sometimes. On a really good day he can but, and he tries real hard, but Gary's stool is very acidy, so you've got to make sure it gets real clean because . . . his skin can break down very quickly, so I have to make sure it's cleaned very well. So he tries, and then I just finish up."

"Is he able to dress himself?"

"He . . . can't dress himself at home. Mostly what he wears is a woman's nightgown with a zipper that goes all the way up because it's the easiest thing on his stomach. There's no pressure on it."

"Is he able to, you said you take him in the bathroom, and is he able to get on and off and take care of his . . ."

"Not usually. No, he needs me, he will call me when he's ready to get off the pot, and I clean him up, and then I, he also has, at this time he's got two bags on him, he's got the bag of TPN that he has on his lap in the morning, and the bag of Dilaudid and those bags can get heavy, so he can't lift them, I need to get the bags and him back to the chair."

"All right, I want to keep you focused . . ., Does he eat a big breakfast?"

"No, Gary is not allowed to eat a big breakfast. The doctors, his GI specialist want him to eat at least eight to ten times a day, little portions like four ounces. If he eats more than that, what happens is he has emesis, which is you heard the doctor say is another word for vomiting. It doesn't sound as bad. And so he's gotten really good, sometimes he will get hungry but, and he pushes himself a little too far and he's throwing up all over the place. If he's not hungry, then I just make coffee and see if he wants any of that and then it's time to start with his medications."

"And is that something quick and easy, how does that go?"

"No. The first medication I give him is normally, if it's been six hours, every six hours I administer Promethazine, which is medication that helps him to stop throwing up. It helps, it doesn't stop it, but it does help the nausea and the vomiting. And after I give him that, I will flush the line again. Now what I have to do is . . ."

"Let me stop you, what is that, flush the line, what does that mean?"

"I'm sorry. Gary has a central line in his chest and it has—like the medical terminology is a double lumen, which means there's two places of access that comes out; one for sixteen hours has TPN in it, the other one has Dilaudid in it. Now when, because there's two accesses, I don't stop the TPN unless it's medically necessary, so I have to stop the Dilaudid and flush the line, I give him his Promethazine, I flush the line again, and then I give him his Protonix. I'm not a registered nurse, so I have to put it in a mini bag, it's a hundred ml's and I have to put it in the bag, mix it up, and then I put a fresh line on and prime it, making sure that there's no air in the line, I hang it up and it takes about fifteen to twenty minutes to go through its cycle. Once it's going through its cycle, I stop it, I flush the line again, and then reconnect his Dilaudid. That's a normal morning up until about ten, eleven o'clock. Depending upon what his sugar is makes a difference on what I give him to eat, or if there's a problem where if it gets, if his sugar gets down into the fifties, Gary has what they call insulin seizures. So what I have to do is be very careful he doesn't have them."

"Is the insulin related to the TPN?"

"Yes. TPN is a big, huge bag that's got all the nutrition, like you have heard from the experts. There's a lot of sugar in that and Gary was never diagnosed as being a diabetic and unfortunately, because he's living on TPN, we'll never know because you have to fast for three days for a physician to probably properly diagnose you as being a diabetic. So what I have to do is I have to put insulin into the TPN to make sure his sugars don't go to high, but I have to make sure his sugars don't go too low. So if his sugar drops, I give him something that will bring it up. If it doesn't bring it up, then after an hour I check his sugar again and if it's still in the fifties, I have to stop the TPN right away and I have to flush the line and I have to start fluids on him, which is just a normal bag of saline, and we would get them in the ER. And that helps just get his body back to normal and brings the sugar back up to where his normal is, which is about a hundred and two or a hundred and sixteen. If it's at that range, then he's doing pretty good, but if it's not then I have to, I have to do what we don't like doing, which is stopping TPN. Unfortunately, a lot of things change in Gary's body, so different things will knock it off when it comes to the TPN, so you have to keep a very close eye on it."

"Where does Gary spend the afternoon?"

"Mostly on the pot. He falls asleep on the toilet a lot and I have to be careful, sometimes I take a pillow in there so he doesn't hurt his neck too much. Or he sits in his chair and falls asleep in his rocker. Because of the way his stomach is he can't lay down flat, it stretches too much and it puts him in too much pain, so he's always, even in the bed, he's in a sitting position. So when he has accidents, it can be sitting there, so I have to make sure that's taken care of."

"You told us about the TPN, is that the mix, set out, tell us what time do you hook the TPN up?"

"Well, we've come up to about noontime, about you know, if it's a Monday per se, this is normally when the nurse would show up, she usually likes to show up between twelve and one o'clock. I have one nurse that comes out, she's there for anywhere from a half hour to an hour and a half, depending upon Gary's needs. She's there, she changes his central line dressing, she draws labs, and she takes his vitals. That's the only nurse I see."

"All week?"

"All week, until the next Monday, unless it's in the ER. If it's not a Monday, then we go through our day, taking care of anything that comes up. When it comes to Gary I'm always thinking okay, let me do this, let me do that, I've got to check this, I'm checking his vitals. And around two or three o'clock I'm pulling the bag of TPN because it's only good for sixteen hours. Now TPN is refrigerated, that's why I'm saying I'm pulling it. I have to take it out of the refrigerator, but I need it to get to room temperature. If I don't let it get to room temperature and it's too cold, it can shock his veins, so you have to make sure it's at room temperature. Now, because it's at home and it's not a hospital setting, there's additives that I have to put in the TPN that they don't normally have to do at the hospital because they have this pharmacy that does it. I don't have a pharmacy that can do that every day. There's four additives that I have to put in the TPN, there's volumes, there's a . . . bottle, and then there's a bottle with insulin. Now the bottle of insulin looks a lot like the other bottle, so you have to be very careful. I take the bottle of insulin out, I draw out how much he's taking, and right now it's only 15 cc's. I put the insulin in. The second thing I do, because if I took that whole bottle and I got confused and I pulled it all out, I would be giving him all that insulin, he would go into a diabetic coma within an hour. So I take that up front, I put it back in the refrigerator so it's separate from everything else. Then I put the other additives in it. After I've added it the last one, I put in a vitamin that's yellow and I use that as a diagram to make sure that I can mix it really well because if it's not yellow at the top, that means I'm not done mixing it, I've got to keep shaking it until I know it's mixed through. If I don't, there could be some insulin down at the bottom and he would get too much too fast, or if you get too much of the other vitamins too fast, so you want to make sure it's mixed really well. Then I have to make sure I connect fresh tubing. . . You have to use new tubing for TPN every time you use TPN, which is every sixteen hours, or for sixteen hours in a twenty-four-hour period, I'm sorry. I put the tubing on, once I put the tubing on, I get my pump out, pour the TPN, because there are different pumps."

"Wait a minute, let me stop you. What do you mean there's different pumps, do you have more than one pump?"

"He's got pump for his Dilaudid that you can see on his lap."

"Right."

"He's got a pump that looks just like that that I use for his TPN. The only difference is the ratio of whatever is programmed into that computer is going into Gary. So I put the battery up, it's a nine-volt battery, and unfortunately there are usually two batteries, so they don't usually last sixteen hours, I'm usually changing them out. All right. Put the battery in and as soon as it goes through its computer stuff it will tell me it's time to prime. There's a back that I connect to it and then I have to lock it. Once I lock it, it tells me make sure the line is clear, and you're ready to prime. So I push the button yes, then I hold the button down and I prime it, and as I'm prim-ing it what you have to do is you have to take the tubing and you have to make sure there's no air in the line, so you're turning it to make sure, you're holding it up so you can make sure that no air stays in the line because you don't want air in your bloodstream. I don't know why, but that's what they told me and I do what I'm told. So I make sure there's no air in Gary's lines. Once it has gone through the system and it goes all the way to the top, after I put those additives in I have a two-hour window to where I have to start the TPN or the bag is no good. If you put a bad bag on Gary it could kill him, so you have to be very careful of making sure you do everything prop-erly and you follow every procedure."

If you put a bad bag on Gary it could kill him.

"Is there a certain speed at which the TPN flows?" Miller asked.

"Yes," Carol said, "there's a ratio and now it just changed so I could be off a little bit on my ratio, the first hour, they call it tapering up, so it runs at a speed of a hundred and ten cc's an hour, which means that is how much of that bag is going into Gary for the first hour. Then it goes down into what they call a, I'm trying to think of what terminology they used, it's just a regular flow, for the next fourteen hours. It's a base rate of like eighty-four, and I could be off on my accounts because they just changed the amounts. That runs for fourteen hours. Then for the last hour, it goes back up to a hundred and ten and it finishes out through the TPN. Now while this is going on within the sixteen hours, you've got a pump that really likes to get annoying and start going off at three or four o'clock in the morning. If you've ever been in the hospital you can hear these pumps in the hospital, they're very sensitive. If there's air in the line, there's backflow, there's a lot of potassium in TPN so Gary's line can clog and if it does you have to stop it, you have to flush the line through and reconnect the TPN and start it back up, or it's no good. So you're having to listen to this, not to mention the fact that it's going to tell you the battery is low halfway through, so you're changing the nine-volt battery also. And then after the TPN is done, off the sixteen hours, I disconnect it, I flush the line and then I heparinize it. I heparinize it so Gary doesn't get blood clots in his line, because the other lines being used, I can only heparinize one line at a time. So I hepa-rinize the line, I wait one to two hours, then I flush the line through and I disconnect the Dilaudid line and I connect it to where the TPN has been running, so I can heparinize that line, because that line has to be heparin-ized too. So I will heparinize that line and then after one to two hours I will transfer it back over. And that's the one that I try to use as much as possible because I have to also give him within this period, I'm giving him Promethazine again, every six hours, and it's not what they call p.r., I think it's p.r.n. is when the patient is asking for it, Gary's is ordered to be given every six hours."

"How do you give that?"

"It's IV, it's just like the Protonix is in a bag, a mini bag, I put it in there, it goes through within fifteen minutes, and it has a line at the top. The lines are only good for twenty-four hours—even in the hospital you can only use the line for twenty-four hours—you have to change it, so I can only use that line for twenty-four hours. So I'm changing that line out."

"And how often do you give that medication, four times a day?"

"The Promethazine is every six hours."

"Okay."

"So whatever that works out to."

"Okay."

"Protonix, I give it to him again at night, he gets forty milligrams of Protonix, which is to get rid of the acid, or to get rid of any other problems that could go on. He's got a lot of things going on in his tummy, there's not much there, but there's a lot going on. So I do that twelve hours later after I've given it to him and by this time, I try to start the TPN right around the same time every day. Sometimes Gary gets really tired and he's like, can you just give me a half hour or can you please start it an hour late? I'm going to give it to him, I'm going to give him that hour. My husband is not asking for much. It may throw my time off, but I don't care, you know? My time is not important because my time is what Gary's needs are. Now if it's a Tuesday instead of a Monday, the only difference in my morning is I'm calling his dietician, there's two of them, and I'm asking what the bloodwork has come back at, because he gets his bloodwork drawn, I'm checking because I need to know if he's low on potassium or magnesium, I cannot do those replacements at home. If he is, I have to take him into the ER, so he does have a lot of trips to the ER, but I have to stay on top of it."

"And I probably cut you off from your evenings. You just described a day."

". . . Yes, and it usually ends for me about two o'clock in the morning."

"Every month you've been doing this twelve months, three hundred and sixty-five days a year?"

"Yes. And if I'm not doing it at home, I'm sleeping on the cot next to him in his bed in the hospital, I don't leave him."

"Other than your son Kenny for that hour, do you get any other long-term relief, from any nurses or any help at all?"

"The only relief I've gotten in the last six months was I was put in the hospital twice and they kept me in there for twenty-four hours and my diagnosis was exhaustion and hypertension."

"You told us about some injuries that you have sustained, is this affecting you physically?"

There was a short sidebar discussion at the bench, during which the judge said, ". . . it's fairly clear, she's already answered that if she's been hospitalized two times for exhaustion, she isn't getting enough sleep."

After that, Miller asked Carol a few questions to firm up his case.

Penhallegon had no questions for her, which was smart. Anything he would ask might strike the jury as beating up on a woman who had been through hell.

Miller rested his case.

When the judge dismissed the jury for the day, she said, "You are a wonderful people who continue to make me happy with your timeliness and your promptness and you're looking so beautiful in that box, I mean, you really do."

# 113

"I was one of the last to testify at the trial," Carol said. "Miller had prepared me the best he could but I think he was a little worried about not being able to shut me up. Was I nervous? No! Was I scared? No! Was I afraid to say the wrong thing? No! Gary and I had the truth on our side. Did I think about what I was going to say? Not really! Do I think I messed up? Yes! At one point I said <u>hospice</u>. If I can remember right, both sides objected. But, before that happened, Miller was asking me about my job history; and, as I started to talk about it, I remembered something Miller had told me which was, we had a choice of having the trial in Baltimore city or Baltimore county.

Miller told us we had a better chance in Baltimore city because the jury would be made up of blue-collar workers. I made a point of always looking at the jury, and I also made a point of bringing up that I was a troubleshooting manager and that meant I would go to stores and clean them up, but the first thing I said was that there are no bad employees, just bad management. Every jury member was shaking their heads *yes*."

# 114

Miller was feeling low.

He believed he had made a strong case and suspected the photographs and video revealing Gary's condition—the internal organs exposed—had been affecting. Still . . .

While he was writing his closing argument at the kitchen table, his son, Jay Jr., who was a teenager, "came in from playing videogames and asked me what I was doing, and I told him. I said, 'I'm going to lose this case.'"

Dad, Jay Jr. said, . . . you've always said one witness doesn't change it, and you just got to figure out how to explain it to the jury. . . . He told me I was the best lawyer . . . And I sat there, and I figured out [how] I was going to reverse it and bring up the fact that here was a doctor who had only been a doctor three months, and *she* knew enough to know that this wasn't Crohn's . . . That's how I played it . . . [And] it worked."

"Peter Angelo's office is a big law office," Carol said. "Most of the office staff never go to see a trial. For the most part the courtroom was empty well until Jay gave his summation."

A dozen people from Angelos's office came to court that day.

"Every one of them came up to Gary and me to wish us good luck," Carol said. "They wanted to show their support for us. I thought this was something they did all the time, however I found out later this was something they never did. Vanessa or Sandy told me she had only been to a courtroom one other time."

Miller gave his closing argument: "Your Honor, may it please the Court. Ladies and gentlemen, Mr. Stern had a right, had an expectation to a diagnosis and treatment for the problem that he presented to the hospital for. Patients have a right, when they go to a hospital, to a diagnosis and a treatment for their problem. Forget you heard so much smoke over this first four days of this May 11th admission. We know when Mr. Stern went in, he had pain in his left upper quadrant that was ten out of ten. We also know that five days later, on the 16th, when he was discharged, it was still eight out of ten.

"The doctors treated Gary for 'a Crohn's flare,' yet there's no explanation for his left upper quadrant pain that is an eight out of ten. If you go back to the calendar, this was the 16th, his pain is still eight out of ten, and that is after being given Dilaudid, and he is discharged. He was discharged, ladies and gentlemen, from Sinai Hospital without a diagnosis for his left upper quadrant pain. He did not have that diagnosis . . . He had classic ulcer pain . . ., and he was discharged from Sinai without a diagnosis. . . .[T]his man just wanted reasonable care, he wanted a reasonable diagnosis for his left upper quadrant pain. Did he get it? . . .Or, did Dr. Heller's decision on the 11th not to do an endoscopy cause Mr. Stern's treatment to head down a road with a catastrophic result?"

Dr. Heller and Dr. Epstein, Miller said, "were the specialists that were brought in, they had the power, they had the expertise to direct Mr. Stern's care. Let's talk about Dr. Heller, because that's the first admission. We know that an endoscopy would have found the ulcer; the real issue is, was there a reason to do an endoscopy? There's no other explanation for this man's pain. None whatsoever. We know that not doing the endoscopy leads to a diagnosis of a Crohn's flare, which leads to no treatment for this ulcer, which leads to this ulcer perforating, which leads to Mr. Stern needing the exploratory surgery. What happens then? [The surgeon] operates and removes a very small section of bowel . . . And speaking of Epstein, next, despite the fact that Mr. Stern is back at the hospital that second time, complaining of the same pain he did on May 11th, and even though he still has this same pain, Dr. Epstein continues with the Crohn's flare diagnosis. He's failed to order IV Protonix, and you have heard that IV Protonix would have healed the ulcer. And we know from Dr. Simon"—an expert witness—"that the perforation that he had in his ulcer led to the destruction of the linkage that he hooked up in his bowel. And all the surgeries that came after that, all resulted from this perforated ulcer . . ."

Gary "thought he was having a heart attack," Miller said. "Here, he told you on the witness stand . . . he hadn't had a problem with his

Crohn's in ten or fifteen years. Where was his prior Crohn's surgery? He pointed down here, and that's where his pain was, years ago. His [current] pain was up here, it felt like he was having a heart attack in his chest, and that's not explainable by a Crohn's flare. Again, this isn't a rare disease, it's an ulcer, something gastros deal with every single day, millions of people have them, and it's such a simple test to check for it . . . [T]hey put the tube down, it takes minutes, minutes. If that endoscopy had been performed, he's not in this wheelchair. With what we have heard from Dr. Langnas," another witness, "forgive me, Gary, it's a death sentence."

## 115

The doctors brought in a consultant, Miller said, "and then they bring in another consultant, and then they bring in another doctor that's going to discharge him. And everybody says, well I only saw him once. It's a reflection of responsibility, that's the age we live in . . . "

Miller continued: "Mr. Penhallegon can spend all the time he wants telling you about his Crohn's, and again, we say so what? He had an ulcer that wasn't diagnosed, it's that simple. He had an ulcer that wasn't diagnosed, and endoscopy would have diagnosed it, and we wouldn't be here today . . . [A]ll of those future complications resulted from a combination of a perforated ulcer, and the anastomosis"—a connection between two separate structures—that [the surgeon]created in that surgery, correct? Correct. They were not caused by his Crohn's Disease, correct? Correct. You agree that the ulcer in combination with the anastomosis, correct, [caused] all those future complications, correct?"

It was Dr. Heller's "job to rule out what was right in front of him," Miller added, "and he never considered peptic ulcer disease. He never did, he testified to that, he never considered it . . . [T]he jury's job is so important, because it is about making people accountable for their actions . . . Can you imagine what would go on in hospitals if there were no system in place to force doctors to take responsibility? If there was no opportunity to make doctors responsible for when they don't do that which the standard of care requires them to do?"

Miller described how every time Gary had a washout the doctors took "a little bit more of his bowel, and a little bit more of his bowel, and each time he lost a little bit more of his bowel, they took a little bit more of Mr. Stern . . . When Ms. Stern got on the stand and told us that he wakes up almost every morning laying in his own feces. Can you imagine the humiliation? When I had an accident in seventh grade, I was sick and I had an accident in my pants, to this day when I see kids in that class, they still make fun of me. And that was one time. I still suffer humiliation from one time. Can you imagine the humiliation that this man suffers daily, waking up every day in his own mess, and not due to anything that he did. That he can't reach around and clean himself up. The simplest things that we take for granted, he can no longer do. Gary . . . can't do what everyone else is blessed and can do, and not because of anything he did. Not because of anything he did. I can't imagine the level of humiliation, I can't imagine the level of mental anguish that these two go through on a daily basis. You know, Gary called her his angel on the stand, and I've seen it myself, for the last couple of weeks. What this lady does for this man, I'll just say that Gary is blessed. When he went country line dancing, and finally didn't stand her up that second time, that was the smartest thing he ever did, because he did marry her, and I would like to think my wife would do this for me, but I just don't know. I don't know. What this lady does, it's unbelievable. And this humiliation, ladies and gentlemen . . . it's every day, it's every day . . . [H]e doesn't have hope that tomorrow might be a different day, because it never is . . . I felt so bad, because Monday, I said, 'How was your weekend?' I asked Carol, 'What did you do?' I said, 'I had steamed crabs, do you like crabs, Gary?' And I had to catch myself. And I thought, he can't enjoy the taste of a steamed crab, or corn on the cob, he can't eat, he can try to get some taste from it, but he can't eat very much of it, because you heard what happens. Cold beer and steamed crabs, I mean, these are things that we take for granted, he can't do . . . We're talking about a man who has his own business, a restaurant, and a bail bonds business, independent, but ironically now he is totally dependent on others. I submit to you, ladies and gentlemen, he is now dependent upon you. Everyone agrees this man is in horrible shape. Everyone agrees it's not his fault. His only hope for any type of future rests now in your hands . . . Ladies and gentlemen, I submit to you, your verdict will give him something he hasn't had for many years, and that's his dignity. Thank you very much."

The jury was faced with two issues:

1. Did the doctors make a mistake?
2. How long would Gary live and how much money would be needed to care for him?

# 116

The day Gary and Carol expected the verdict—September 2, 2015—Miller was nervous, Gary was stressed, and Carol was intense.

"I knew we had won," Carol said, "but I had no idea how much."

The judge called everyone into the courtroom. Miller told them to move to where he was sitting. Carol pushed Gary's wheelchair and stood behind him with both of her hands on Gary's shoulders. David was standing behind them with his hand on Gary's back.

"Members of the jury," the clerk said, "have you agreed upon a verdict?"

All the jurors said Yes.

"And your foreperson shall speak for you?" the clerk said.

All the jurors said Yes.

"Madame Foreperson," the clerk said, "could you please stand? In the case of Gary B. Stern and Carol Bishop-Stern versus Todd Heller, M.D., and Steven Epstein, M.D. . . . do you find by a preponderance of the evidence that defendant Todd Heller, M.D., deviated from the standard of care in his treatment of the plaintiff, Gary B. Stern, yes or no?"

The foreperson said, "Yes."

"As to B," the clerk asked, "do you find by a preponderance of the evidence that Dr. Heller's breach of the ethical standard of care was a proximate cause of injury and/or damage to Gary B. Stern, yes or no?"

The foreperson said, "Yes."

"As to Question 2, as to defendant Steven Epstein, M.D.," the clerk said, "do you find by a preponderance of the evidence that defendant Steven

Epstein, M.D. deviated from the standard of care in his treatment of the plaintiff, Gary B. Stern, yes or no?"

The foreperson said, "Yes."

"As to B," the clerk said, "do you find by a preponderance of the evidence that Dr. Epstein's breach of the ethical standard of care was a proximate cause of injury and/or damage to Gary B. Stern, yes or no?"

The foreperson said, "Yes."

"As to Question 3," the clerk said, "what amount of damages do you award plaintiff Gary B. Stern for A, past medical expenses?"

"One million, ninety-seven thousand, thirty-two dollars and ninety-eight cents," the foreperson said.

"As to B," the clerk asked, "future medical and life care expenses?"

"Fourteen million, two hundred seventy-seven thousand, one hundred and sixty dollars," the foreperson said.

"As to C," the clerk asked, "noneconomic damage?"

"Eight million dollars," the foreperson said.

"What amount of damages do you award the plaintiff Gary B. Stern and Carol Stern for loss of consortium?" the clerk asked.

"Five million dollars," the foreperson said.

Carol leaned over to tell Gary, "We did it," but Gary was crying so hard, he didn't hear the amount.

The jury members were dismissed. Carol gazed at them. Not one them said anything to Gary and Carol, but a couple of them were smiling, the rest of them were crying.

"How much?" Gary had collected himself. "How much?"

He wanted it to be enough to take care of Carol for life.

"I thought Jay was going to explode," Carol said. "All I could do was to thank God."

Miller repeated what Carol had said: "We did it."

Gary repeated what he had asked: "How much?"

"You didn't hear it?" Miller asked.

Miller asked Warshaw, "What was the total?"

"Hold on," Mike said, "I'm still adding it up."

"Did you hear how much?" Gary asked Carol.

"No, baby," Carol said, "I'm not sure, but we won. They believed you. We just needed to tell the truth."

"I added it up three times," Mike said.

$27,500,000.00

"How much?" Miller asked.

"What?" Gary asked.

Miller asked Mike to add it up again.

"$27,500,000.00."

"That's the most anyone has ever been awarded for a single case in Baltimore," Miller said.

"How much?" Miller asked.

"What?" Curr asked.

Miller asked Mike to add it up again.

"$22,500,000.00."

"That's the most anyone has ever been awarded for a single case in Baltimore," Miller said.

# Part Four

---

# Grief

## 117

"I thought that any downside at all would be overridden by [Gary's and Carol's] personalities," Miller said. "I thought they were the reason we hit so big. I think the jury felt that Carol . . . had dedicated her life, and the defense took the approach that they don't need a nurse to come in, his wife can change his TPN. And even though she was doing it, should [we] continue to make his wife take care of him 24/7? That's what we're asking? You know, it was just awful."

There was a tremendous amount of publicity.

"Write ups in different legal publications . . . Professionally, it was a big feather in my cap." But "for the client's perspective," because Maryland has a cap on what you can recover for pain and suffering, the judge had to strike nine million," from the ten million for "pain and suffering."

"For thirty years," Miller said, "all I've ever done is represent victims, and this case is the ultimate case of satisfaction for someone like me . . . to know that after this case was over, all that hard work, now these people really will have a chance at a life where they . . . can hire somebody to take care of him, she really can get a new van with a wheelchair lift . . . All those . . . things that I was asking the jury for, they were really going to be able to get, and that was overwhelming satisfaction. I mean, overwhelming satisfaction. I think about it right now, and I can get that feeling in my stomach all over again."

The law is not always about justice, it's about what you can get away with, about who tells a better story. There's a difference between God's Law and Man's Law. Under Man's Law, justice is not always done. In Gary's and Carol's case, Miller believed that God's Law and Man's Law coincided. Justice was done.

"I've tried a lot of cases in my career, and I've . . . lost cases that I never should have lost, I've won cases that I never should have won. I've won cases because I was the better arguer. This case . . . every once in a while, the system works exactly the way it's supposed to." Gary's and Carol's "lives were changed by that result."

Still—Miller knew—"the ending is tragic, I wish [Gary] was here, I really do."

"Most people were amazed," by the verdict, "because it was not a case . . . I was talking . . . up a lot."

Miller's friends and family didn't see Gary's and Carol's case as significant; another run-of-the-mill medical malpractice case.

Some of them told Miller, that they didn't even know he was trying a big case . . .

But "when they heard the details . . .," Miller said, "it was overwhelming. Everybody was overwhelmingly happy for this couple who had faced such tragedy."

# 118

Mike Warshaw took Carol's suitcase. Miller wheeled Gary along the sidewalks. Carol walked next to the wheelchair and held Gary's hand.

By the time they got to Miller's office, Gary was so excited Carol was worried he would have a seizure. Carol took him back to the hotel and gave him his medication. They had dinner. Gary got out of his clothes and slept for an hour. When he woke up, they called everyone to tell them the news.

The next day, Jeanette called Carol to say it didn't look good for Willem.

Before Gary got sick, Gary and Carol would meet Jeanette and Willem for dinner every time they came into town—about once a month. After Gary got sick, Willem refused to have their dinners until Gary could eat again. When they got back from Cleveland to Baltimore, the dinners resumed.

During the trial, Carol said, "We called Mom and Pop every night to tell them what happened," Carol said. "After the first week Mom was taking all the calls from us"—which seemed odd. The second week of Willem skipping the calls, Gary asked to talk to him. Jeanette said he had gone to bed, but they knew that couldn't be true because Jeanette needed Willem's help getting herself into bed.

The next day, on September 3, Jeanette told Carol that Willem was in the hospital. Willem didn't want Gary to know. He didn't want to add to Gary's worries.

A few days later, when it didn't look as if Willem was getting better and when Gary was having a good day, Carol told him. "We never had a chance to celebrate the verdict."

They had planned to go to a casino. Instead, Gary and Carol packed and went to West Virginia.


# 119

On September 5, Gary and Carol arrived in West Virginia.

September 7 was Gary's birthday. Two days later, September 9, Willem died. On the 19, Gary and Carol went back to North Carolina.

Gary and Carol were so busy that neither of them paid attention when Kenny warned them that all the walls in the Pinch Gut house were red.

"Boy, did we find out how red they were when we got home," Carol said.

Two o'clock in the afternoon. They opened the car door and were swarmed with mosquitoes. Carol and Kenny scrambled Gary into the house, waving away the bugs.

"It was an invasion of the mosquitoes," Carol said.

Ducking the bugs, they slammed the door behind them, and looked at the walls. Which were, as Kenny had said, red. Not pink. Not vermillion. Not rust. Not reddish, rosy, or off-red.

Red.

Bright red.

Kenny was killing mosquitoes that had flown into the house, swatting ten to twenty at a time. There were dead mosquitoes all over the walls.

The red walls.

Next to the house was farm land. Carol and Kenny spent three days killing mosquitoes and cleaning off the walls; then, the farmer sprayed his crops. Whatever he used turned the walls from red speckled with dead bugs to black.

"So we had red-and-black buggy walls," Carol said, "and I needed Gary in a sterile environment."

Carol needed to move Gary, and fast.

"I couldn't let Gary stay there," Carol said. "It would have killed him."

Carol did the only thing she could think of.

"I moved us to a hotel," she said.

They went to the Hilton Garden Inn in Kitty Hawk, near where the Wright Brothers flew their first airplanes.

# 120

In 2012, in Baltimore, Carol had opened an account at Wells Fargo.

Jay Miller—Gary and Carol's attorney—needed Gary to sign and notarize papers, but Gary was in no condition to go to the bank. Carol called Lee, her Wells Fargo banker, who made a phone call to a branch in the Outer Banks, which arranged for Chad Weeks to go to the hotel with notary Ann Shepherd.

Gary was very sick. They didn't stay long.

"Sick or not," Carol said, "Gary was a great judge of character."

Gary wanted to like Chad, but Chad was a banker, and Gary's father had imbued in Gary a distrust of bankers.

"When Gary met Chad," Carol said, "it was one of the few times Gary was not put off by a banker."

Chad even helped Carol set up her GPS, which had a male voice.

"I am not going to have any other man but Gary tell me what to do," Carol said, "so Chad changed the GPS to a woman's voice."

After the notary was done, Carol and one of her sisters were trying to find a place to rent. Kenny stayed at Pinch Gut to pack up and take care of the dogs.

Gary was getting sicker, and so was Carol, who wasn't sleeping or eating. They both ended up in the Outer Banks ER. Gary had an infection. Carol suffered from exhaustion. The doctor kept them in the hospital for two days.

# 121

They found a rental on Craigslist, one that had been posted just minutes before she saw it.

Gary and Carol loved the place, Carol a little more than Gary because it had a long driveway, a wraparound porch (a feature Jeanette had loved), and was on a canal.

"And that's what put us, on September 1, 2015, on 116 Duck Woods Drive," Carol said.

Gary, Carol, and Kenny spent the first month trying to settle in and get organized. Gary could eat, but he couldn't get any nutrition from what he ate, so he had to stay on the TPN. Carol called Mason at Equinox, where he got his TPN, and arranged to get everything Gary needed.

Gary cooked lamb, standing at the stove, hooked up to his IV.

"When he peered into the oven," Robert said, "he almost put his IV in with the lamb."

When Gary felt good, he wanted to eat.

"He was always sneaking food," Robert said.

# 122

Carol hired two nurses—Janet Jordan ("Miss Janet" Gary and Carol called her) and Meredith Lasko ("Kelly" everyone called her)—who came in every day but Sundays, each working an eight-hour shift. Gary was cared for sixteen hours a day.

At first, it was hard to have the help, because Gary didn't want anyone else in the house.

"He had problems giving up control," Carol said. "But we both knew it's what we needed."

Miss Janet, who was an RN (registered nurse) from Quality Staffing, started working with Gary on November 4, 2015. She was a tenth-generation Acadian French Canadian (her maiden name is Arsenault) who grew up in Ottawa. She kept her first husband's [Tommy's] name, because it was "less complicated when it comes to all of the paperwork regarding resident alien [status]."

"I wanted to work with the dying patients," Miss Janet said.

She had been influenced by Elizabeth Kubler-Ross's book *On Death and Dying.*

"My father had lung cancer," she said, "and I hung about quite a bit in the hospital, and the chaplain and the nurses encouraged me, and said . . . 'You have a gift for this'. . . A year later, I signed up for nursing school, and I graduated three years later," when she was forty-three.

On a vacation in the Outer Banks, she had met a man she liked, "so," she said, "I moved down here . . .. Sadly, that didn't work out well, but, after seven years, I moved on, and now I'm married to my wonderful husband of twenty, almost twenty-five years, Tex Gallop," a captain on the Hatteras Ferry," and a fifth-generation Outer Banks fisherman.

Her father and brother were spiritualists, which influenced her, part of the reason she had worked twice in Kolkata at Mother Teresa's House for the Dying. Once a year, usually in February to March, Miss Janet went to Antigua to volunteer at a hospice named St. John's.

Miss Janet was a city girl, "an inner-core-area person . . . So the Outer Banks was quite different for me," but, she said, "What I require in my life is variety."

She had taken care of ventilator-dependent children, worked in a nursing home for many years in various capacities, worked as a hospital nurse, and was a private duty nurse. But, she said, "nothing ever came close to Gary."

She had not spoken with Carol before she showed up at Carol's front door.

"That was quite an astounding day," Miss Janet said. "Carol met me at the door"—Gary and Carol had just moved in—"and the first thing . . . I had to go meet Gary, [who] . . . was . . . sitting in his room, in his chair, and he was very . . . cautious, personable, [but] not particularly open."

She could tell Gary was a very private person.

She had never met anyone with Carol's focus.

"It was obsessive," she said. ". . . I thought, 'Oh gosh, what's with this?'"

She called Carol The Interceptor, because "She intercepted death, okay?"

Miss Janet quoted Emily Dickinson's "Because I could not stop for Death—He kindly stopped for me . . ."

She did her nursing assessment.

Gary's "skin [is] warm and dry, [his] pupils are equal and reactive to light . . ."

But she had to do it quickly. Gary was impatient.

She checked the two pumps—TPN and pain medicine—going into Gary's central line, "directly into his heart."

Gary's room was, she thought, "set up like a little hospital."

Carol had plastic storage bins: Heparin syringes, normal saline syringes, all the different medications. Quickly, she realized that Gary's mental health was as important as his physical health—and, Carol reminded her, his spiritual health and his emotional health.

"Wow," Miss Janet said, "you want to talk about . . . taking care of somebody holistically . . ."

Carol went through the whole drill: what Gary needed, what she needed to help what Gary needed.

"She spoke to me about the dog," Miss Janet said, "and his very specific barking."

On her way to the laundry room to do a wash, "I could look at Gary," without being intrusive. "I would . . . glance in" and "eyeball his chest" the same way she used to with ventilator-dependent children.

"The first day," Miss Janet continued, "I'm sitting over there on this little bench."

"I'm going to try and lie down," Carol said.

"Obviously," Miss Janet said, "she had not had any sleep at all . . . This was 24/7, okay? Talk about sleep deprivation, wow."

On Miss Janet's first night helping to take care of Gary, she heard someone call.

"Here I am," Miss Janet said, sounding like Moses answering the Lord.

Of course, Gary was calling Carol.

"Her first night at the house with us was a night I won't ever forget," Carol said. "I don't think she will either."

For the previous three days, Gary had been having a bad time. In three days, Carol as usual managed only three hours of sleep.

Gary could drift off, but couldn't go into a deep sleep, because when he did he would go to the bathroom.

"Miss Janet could tell we both needed sleep," Carol said. "She didn't say much."

She just figured out Gary and Carol and their routines. After Carol showed her around, she gave her instructions: what to do if she saw anything wrong with Gary.

Gary was sitting in his chair in the bedroom. Carol had given him his medication and started his TPN. Miss Janet was sitting on the window seat that had a view of the kitchen. Carol had laid down in the bed next to Gary.

"I have no idea how long I was asleep," Carol said, "but I do know I was in a deep sleep."

Carol doesn't know what woke her.

"It was like someone shook me or something," Carol said, "but no one was in the bedroom."

Not even Gary.

Carol jumped out of bed and ran into the kitchen.

"Gary was at the sink," Carol said, "but it wasn't really Gary."

Sometimes Gary seemed to be in an alternate reality. He did things, but didn't know he was doing them.

From where Miss Janet sat, she couldn't see Gary, who was wandering around with his IV pole. He went into the living room, where Miss Janet was sitting, facing away from him.

"He was a bit growly," Miss Janet said. "He wanted to wake Carol up. Remember, he says 'Carol' every twelve minutes. 'Carol. Carol. Carol.' He's either asking her something or wanting to know where she is."

Gary continued his wandering, ending at the kitchen sink, where he turned on the water tap.

"Carol comes flying out of the bedroom," Miss Janet said, "because she senses these things."

Instead of running the water into the sink, Gary had put that faucet over to the side of the sink. The water overflowed onto the floor.

"He had no idea he's doing it," Miss Janet said, "because all of his medicine levels were off."

Butchy was nowhere around, so he hadn't alerted Carol, Miss Janet said.

Carol called Kenny, who said, "Mom, I'm on my way."

Miss Janet thought Gary's confusion was due to electrolyte imbalances.

"Gary gets confused when all his numbers are off," Carol said.

Water was still pouring all over the floor. Carol wanted to stop him, but she didn't want to startle him because he might fall and get hurt. Gary walked into the living room and started to light his central line on fire. First, water. Then, fire.

Carol had to stop him. He got upset.

Miss Janet was cleaning up the water.

Gary disconnected his TPN and pain pump and was looking for another lighter.

"Every time I stopped him," Carol said, "he got more and more upset."

By the time Kenny arrived—within five minutes—Carol had eased Gary, who still had his lighter, into the shower.

Kenny told Carol to get out of the shower.

"I've got this," Kenny said. "You need to go get cleaned up."

Miss Janet had finished cleaning up the mess in the kitchen and living room.

"Is it always like this?" she asked.

"We have our moments," Carol said.

"How did you know something was wrong," Miss Janet asked. "I was sitting right here, and I didn't see it."

"I just knew Gary needed me," Carol said. "I don't know how to explain it."

"But," Miss Janet said, "you were sleeping."

"It's not the first time," Carol said, "and unfortunately it will happen again. But I can always call my son. He's always close by."

Kenny had settled Gary in his chair. Soon, Gary was asleep.

"Mom," Kenny said, "you can come in and reconnect everything now."

That night Carol got at most half-an-hour of sleep—not unusual. Miss Janet was getting ready to go home.

"I'm driving along down the street," Miss Janet said, "and I'm saying to myself, *Wow. Did I just see that? Wow. Wow.* I remember thinking" that's where God wanted "me to be . . . *Okay, okay Lord, whatever the need is. . . I don't know what I can do here, but You'll help me figure it out.*"

She could not believe what Carol was doing for Gary or how sick Gary was.

"When I was doing my clinical," Miss Janet said, "a patient whom I had been with all day . . ." would ask her, "Are you back tomorrow?"

If she were lacking confidence, she would think the question meant, *Oh, gosh, he hates me, I didn't take good care of her today, she's hoping I'm not going to be back tomorrow.* As her confidence grew, she no longer beat herself up. If someone asked, "Are you back tomorrow?" she figured it meant the opposite of her fears: *They wanted to make sure I would be continuing to take care of them.*

# 123

Gary opened up with Miss Janet when he was humming "Hava Nagila," an Israeli folk song, and Miss Janet, who was folding laundry, started singing along.

"His head snapped around," Miss Janet said.

"Do you know that song?" he asked.

"Well, yeah," Miss Janet said.

She didn't say, "Doesn't everyone?"

Gary talked to Miss Janet "about being Jewish . . . The next thing I told him [was] how much I loved the movie *Yentl.*'" Oddly, Miss Janet said, she had watched a Barbra Streisand television special two nights earlier, during which Streisand sang, "Papa Can You Hear Me," from *Yentl.*

"Wasn't that [song] wonderful," Gary said. "He was crying."

"Don't hold it in," Miss Janet told Gary, "just let it out. It's okay."

Miss Janet had two albums of *Yentl*—she didn't know why, very much like Gary having two of things—which she played on an old record player she bought for $25 at a thrift store.

"When I asked Gary if I should play the song, he said no. 'That's okay,' I said, "another time.'"

At one point she brought the record and record player over, but Gary wasn't up to listening to it. Too emotional.

There was another "intense moment . . ."

It happened on one of the rare times Carol went out to the store. Gary stood at the mantel, staring at the picture of his parents' wedding. He told Miss Janet he hadn't seen it before; Kenny had just put it up there.

Gary "put his hand on his mother . . . "

He stood like that for fifteen minutes.

Miss Janet was busy at the sink, but she could tell Gary was teary.

"I miss my mom," Gary said.

Miss Janet put her arms around him.

"Gary was . . . shaky," Miss Janet said, "so I helped him back to his room. And then he told me about his dad. He knew his father loved him, but I don't think his father was . . . demonstrative . . . He remembered that as a child, being in the hospital with his Crohn's . . . "

"My dad used to come into the hospital after working hard, hard, hard all day," Gary said.

# 124

Kelly—a Level Two Certified Nursing Assistant (CNA), a caretaker for seventeen years—took the other shift.

Her father owned a string of water sports businesses: jet skis, wave runners, parasailing.

When the weather was too cold or windy for water sports, they gave people tours of Carova to see the last of the Spanish wild mustangs.

There are only seventy left out of a hundred and seventy-seven, descendants of horses that came over with the conquistadors or, later, imported work horses. Some swam to shore from the shipwrecks.

"We would [lead] the horse tour riding down the beach," Kelly said. "My favorite tour guides are retired Coast Guard . . . You would be going at the same speed as the horses and the dolphins or the whales, and it's pretty cool to see."

Kelly and her brother own a piece of property on Penny's Hill, next to Jockey's Ridge.

"It's the second largest sand dune on the East Coast," Kelly said. "It moves about five feet a year . . . [T]here's a whole town from the 1800s buried underneath [the sand]. [It's] called Seagull."

A few years ago, in October, "one of our tour guides found a Spanish doubloon up there from 1535," Kelly said. "My brother Vance got so geeked out . . . he went out and bought the best metal detector money could buy."

He found five doubloons.

"Some people search their whole lives for one," Kelly said. "He found three silver and two silver and gold . . . You could see the Spanish cross, the writing. . . It it was perfectly preserved. . . They were all in different locations . . . ."

But the locations change because the land changes.

About one island, Kelly said, "Google it and look how much the storms have changed it in the last three years . . . [We're] fighting Mother Nature, which is ridiculous."

Kelly's first impressions of Gary and Carol: "It was apparent right away that [Carol was] . . . the most devoted wife anyone could have. Carol was sleep-deprived, exhausted, she would . . . sleep thirty minutes at a time, and she . . . was so in tuned to [Gary], they used to joke that Carol was an honorary R.N. . . I was sad that this had happened to them."

Kelly was struck by "how thin Gary was . . . He was so frail—and he was in . . . the kitchen, fussing around, doing something, and . . ." Not exactly sneaking food, because, Kelly explained, "there were no dietary restrictions."

They were trying to make Gary "happy and comfortable."

At first, Gary was "standoffish," Kelly said. "[He didn't want anybody here but Janet [the other nurse], so me, being the new person, it was" awkward.

"We talked about him being a bounty hunter," Kelly said. "I tried to find something that . . . he was excited about."

A bounty hunter—"that's . . . how he opened up to me, telling me about that."

Kelly said she always tried to find something she could use to bond with her patients.

"I knew Carol loved me," Kelly said. "Even though I thought that Gary liked me, he always wanted Janet. Carol told me once that Janet reminded him of someone" named Vashtella, "the woman that used to take care of him when he was a child, when his parents were out of town."

# 125

---

Gary wanted to charter a plane—"a train," Carol corrected—and go to Las Vegas to a boxing match.

"He was really excited about this trip," Kelly said.

"We'd also see the Grand Canyon," Carol said.

Gary had mentioned he had flown over the Grand Canyon many times, but he wanted to see it on the ground.

"I wanted to give him something to look forward to," Carol said.

Gary sent Kelly out to get Carol's favorite roses, her yellow roses.

"I thought how sweet that this man, in the middle of all this going on," made sure he got his wife flowers, Kelly said. "He snuck me some money and sent me on my way" to the florist.

"Carol opened up to me about how they got down here and everything that had happened," Kelly said, "trying to share some of her history in the hospital, and how she pioneered these techniques, and showed me a picture of them before Gary got sick. And I remember thinking, *I would have loved to have met them before Gary got sick, because he looks like a badass . . .* There was just something about him." He struck Kelly as having "a little hustler in him.. Maybe that was part of his job as a bail bondsman, bounty hunter, but he was . . . quick-witted, and I used to think *Man, they must have been quite the power couple before this happened to him.*"

A "glamorous couple."

Kelly knew what Gary did was "a hard line of work, all your phone calls come . . . in the middle of the night."

Kelly imagined Gary "waiting at his bar for a call, to get some person out of jail, I just thought man, that must have been . . . crazy, he's like [an upscale version of] "Dog the Bounty Hunter."

To the end —Kelly said—Gary "was trying to . . . do romantic things for Carol."

One time, Gary asked Kelly to get lamb chops because Carol loved them.

"He really was so sick at that point," Kelly said, "he couldn't do anything but just send us out to do things for him," but he always made sure he had loving surprises for Carol.

# 126

Dr. Kindall was Gary's GI in Greenville, about two hours away from where they were living. He had worked with Dr. Kareem when they were both in Pennsylvania—which made things a little less complicated, which was also true of Gary's dietitian. Equinox was sending Gary's TPN to the house. A nurse came every Monday for about fifteen minutes. There was a fire station on the street. For emergencies, Carol gave them a copy of Gary's medical condition and medication so they would know what to do when—if? — Carol called.

Carol took Gary to Greenville once every six to eight weeks to see his GI doctor and his dietitian and once a month to see his primary doctor. Pain medication was still a problem, because nothing stayed in his body long enough to take effect. The same with his seizure medication, and Gary was having from four to ten seizures a week. They spent a lot of time in the ER.

"Unfortunately, when most doctors in the ER in North Carolina saw how much pain medication Gary was getting, they assumed he was addicted," Carol said. An old story for them. "But after ten minutes of explaining, they would come around and help. Some. Not all."

Given the procedures Gary had been through, David thought, did it even matter if Gary had become addicted?

Out of Gary's earshot, Carol told the nurse "when I put my finger up, give him a placebo."

"There were times where Gary would get anxious and wouldn't let the medication work for him," Carol said, "so I would have the nurse just do a double flush. Gary would think he was getting medication when he really wasn't. And it relaxed his mind enough so the medication he *did* have inside him could work a little better. That sounds rotten, but I did have to worry about him getting too much medicine."

"I know when I'm getting a placebo," Gary told David. "Carol thinks that she's getting the better of me, but she's not."

"Dr. Karen McPherson had a special way with Gary," Carol said. "Every time we left her office, Gary was happy and wanted to keep trying to gain weight. We would always go to Kentucky Fried Chicken and get two drumsticks and mashed potatoes."

Carol would drive to a spot on the beach. Gary watched the waves and ate his chicken, in the van. They talked about the day they would sit on the beach and picnic."

But that day never came.

# 127

Gary had been in the North Carolina hospitals so many times that Carol lost track. Usually, he went in because of infections, blockages, seizures, iron infusions, and dehydration.

"The one thing I heard more than anything else, was that Gary had only twenty-four hours to live," Carol said. "The next day Gary would be sitting up, ready to be discharged."

Carol was hospitalized again for exhaustion. This time she wouldn't let them put her in the hospital unless they put Gary there, too. The hospital staff put a note on Carol's door to come in only twice a day, so she could rest. She only wanted them to let her know that Gary was all right.

She woke up twenty-seven hours later. They went back home.

Another time, Gary came into the kitchen and said, "Did you put the girls' hamburger meat in the refrigerator."

"What are you talking about?" Kimberly, Carol's daughter, said.

"The patties that you made," Gary said.

"Gary," Kimberly said, "that was yesterday."

He yelled at himself for being so out of it. He took his bag and his IV and walked away.

"I looked at Mom," Kimberly said, "and asked, 'What happened?'"

"He's embarrassed because his, of his mind, you know, everything is jumbled together," Carol said.

# 128

Gary was in his rocking chair in the bedroom. One of Carol's sisters was in the shower. Carol—also in the bedroom—was trying to corral the dogs, when Butchy stared at Gary and then looked at Carol, crying. That meant Gary was about to have a seizure. Carol shouted for her sister.

Gary jerked his head up to the right and said, "Carol, Carol, Carol," and then "Oh, no. Oh, no. Oh, no."

Carol's sister ran out of the bathroom, dripping wet. She was on one side of the bed, Gary and Carol were on the other side.

"What do I do?" Carol's sister asked. "What do I do?"

This happened on October 1 at 9:30 a.m.

In his fit, Gary had broken some of his teeth. Carol put her fingers in Gary's mouth to scoop them out. She was afraid that if he swallowed his teeth it might cause another fistula.

"Call 911," Carol told her sister, who did.

"My brother-in-law is having a seizure," she said into the phone. "116 Duck Woods Drive." Carol's sister passed on the 911 instructions to Carol. "Make sure he doesn't hit his head and make sure his doesn't choke."

"Tell her he has a short gut," Carol said. "He broke his teeth, and I can't let him swallow them."

Carol's sister told the 911 operator and then said to Carol, "She said that if we have dogs, we need to put them up."

"You can put Zenny and Princie in the bathroom," Carol said, "but Butchy won't go."

"We have a dog that will not leave Gary's side when his having a seizure," Carol's sister told 911. Then to Carol: "Will Butchy let the paramedics take care of Gary?"

Carol's sister got off the phone and was putting Zenny and Princess in the bathroom when they heard the sirens.

"I don't have any clothes on," she said.

"Put on a towel," Carol said. "At least . . ."

The paramedics came in and started working on Gary. Carol's sister got dressed. Carol and her sister followed the paramedics to the Outer Banks Hospital.

Carol and her sister were in the room with Gary, who was out of it for half hour or so. The doctor told Carol not to worry about Gary swallowing his teeth.

"He could get a fistula," Carol said.

"A what?" The doctor asked.

Carol repeated, "A fistula."

The doctor looked as if he didn't know what a fistula was.

"A hole in his intestines," Carol said.

"That shouldn't happen," the doctor said.

"Shit," Carol thought, "another idiot doctor."

The doctor came in and said Gary could go back home.

Hungry, Carol ordered from Grits Grill, the restaurant next to the hospital. She and her sister got into the van, Gary in the back seat, Carol's sister in the front. Carol went into the restaurant to pick up their food. When she got back into the van and put the bag of food down on the floor, Gary had another seizure.

"Gary only called my name once," Carol said. "It was one of his worse seizures."

It took two weeks for Carol to remember what happened.

"Here goes," she said. "I turned around to look at Gary. His head jerked. His eyes rolled back. His body fell to the side of his chair. He was drooling on both sides of his mouth. He was choking. He turned red, then blue."

Carol's sister couldn't do anything. She didn't know how.

The hospital was right next door, but they were in another parking lot. Carol didn't know if she should drive out of the restaurant parking lot and to the hospital emergency room entrance or to get in the back of the van and give Gary CPR.

"I had to pick fast," Carol said.

She slammed the van into reverse and tore out of the restaurant backwards, her hand on the horn, and backwards on the wrong side of the road, swung into the emergency room entrance, her hand still on the horn.

No one came out of the hospital.

Carol told her sister to keep her hand on the horn.

By the time Carol got out of the van and opened the back door, LPNs arrived with a wheelchair.

"But they just stood there saying 'what do I do?' Like my sister," Carol said.

"Help me get him out," Carol said. "He's not breathing."

"Maybe I should get a gurney," one of the nurses said.

"Fuck the gurney," Carol said.

"I'm not sure how to move him," the nurse said. "He's connected to his pump."

"Fuck it," Carol said. "Just stand there."

Carol disconnected Gary's pump, prayed *Lord, give me strength*, picked up Gary's shaking blue body, and put him in the wheelchair.

The LPNs took Gary inside.

"I couldn't help myself," Carol said. "I lost it."

Her body started shaking. She started crying hysterically. Some nurses put her in a wheelchair.

As they were rolling her into the hospital, Carol's voice told her, *Don't lose it. Gary needs you.*

"I snapped out of it," Carol said.

Carol went into Gary's room, which was crowded with nurses and doctors, working on Gary.

After twenty minutes Gary was stabilized. In his happy place.

Carol went outside for a cigarette.

"Boy," Carol said, "that didn't work."

Carol's thoughts were racing. *What just happened? Why did Gary have another seizure? Does he have an infection? What the hell is wrong with this hospital? Why are they treating Gary like shit? They're treating him like nothing is wrong and his life doesn't matter. That's exactly what they're doing. Bullshit. No one treats Gary like that.*

Carol needed to fix this, and now.

*What to do? What to do? Patient advocate.*

She had just lit her third cigarette, which she flipped onto the ground as if she were setting off a bomb.

*Well,* Carol thought. *Maybe I was.*

She stormed into the hospital and confronted the woman behind the desk who was volunteering.

"I need to see the patient advocate," Carol said.

"Can I help you with something?" the volunteer asked.

"Yes," Carol said, "you can get me a patient advocate."

Carol was sure she could see how mad she was because she didn't say another word. She pick up the phone and called.

"About five minutes went by," Carol said. "This was not good for me. No, this was not good for them."

Finally, a patient advocate—a woman—came out.

"Are you the head patient advocate?" Carol asked.

No, she said, but I am a patient advocate.

"Not good enough. Get me the head patient advocate."

Can I ask what it's about?

"No, just get me the head patient advocate."

"I didn't sound very nice," Carol admitted. "Well, I wasn't very nice. This hospital wasn't taking care of Gary right and I was going to fix that."

As the head patient advocate—a man—came down the hall, they checked each other out like two gunfighters.

He introduced himself and asked what he could do.

"We need to go someplace to talk," Carol said.

He pointed at some chairs and asked, "How about over there?"

"No," Carol said. "I don't want anyone to hear what I have to say. Let me rephrase that. You don't want anyone else to hear what I have to say."

One of Carol's sisters saw Carol and a man she didn't know walking through the emergency room. She could tell Carol was mad. She headed over to Carol and the patient advocate, who was saying, "How about the Chapel?"

*What I have to say shouldn't be said in a Chapel,* Carol said to herself. *Okay, what I have to say shouldn't have to be said at all.*

"Okay," Carol told the patient advocate. "Let's go into the Chapel."

Inside the Chapel, the head patient advocate said, Tell me what's going on.

"Let me start by saying that in the last five years my husband has been in the hospital for 85 percent of the time," Carol said. "In more than ten hospitals, and this hospital is in the running of the three worst hospitals, and it's a close race."

Carol's sister started to say something.

Carol shot her a look.

"Shut up," Carol told her sister. "I will take care of this."

To the head patient advocate, Carol said, "My husband has been a very sick man for years now. The doctors and the nurses at this hospital are such idiots. They have absolutely no medical knowledge. The doctor [taking caring of Gary] didn't even seem to know what a fistula is. The only thing they seem to know is how to treat a sunburn or a shark bite, and even then that patient would probably die of an infection. My husband has been at this hospital many times, and the only thing they seem to care about is how much pain medication he is getting. Well, I stopped that by getting a pain pump."

"Carol," Carol's sister said. "Your blood pressure. Calm down."

"I can't calm down," Carol snapped. "This is my husband I'm talking about. I will not calm down. He will be treated right."

Carol glanced at the door, through the glass panel at the top. A police officer was looking at Carol, who waved him in.

"You should hear this, too," Carol said to the cop. "If your loved ones get sick, don't bring them here unless you want them to die."

"Calm down," one of Carol's sisters interrupted. "You're going to have a heart attack."

"God is not going to let me have a heart attack here," Carol said. "These doctors would put a Band-Aid on my knee. God wants me to take care of Gary."

Carol was pacing with her hands on her hips.

To the policeman, Carol repeated, "Don't let your loved ones come here."

Carol looked at the head patient advocate, who said, Please, tell me what happened.

"My husband had a Grand Mal seizure," Carol said. "It was so bad he broke his teeth and was swallowing them. My husband only has seventeen inches of his intestines left. And if he gets another fistula, he's going to die. I'm not going to let that happen. The doctor is so nonchalant about it, he sent us home. We only made it to the next parking lot before he had another one, which was worse than the first. I don't understand how or why he had a second one, but I need to know so it doesn't happen again."

I will go find out, the head patient advocate said. What else can I do?

"I want it in my husband's records," Carol said, "and the first thing is that he be treated like a patient, not a drug addict. This hospital has no idea how to treat patients. He's to be treated like a king. If not, I will own this hospital, and I will fire everyone here. And don't think I can't. You would be surprised what I can do when it comes to my husband."

After a moment, Carol added, "And I want someone in my husband's room at all times until we leave."

<u>Okay</u>, the head patient advocate said, <u>I will go make sure all of this is</u> <u>taken care of. I will be right back.</u>

"My sister will be with Gary," Carol said. "I'm going outside to have a cigarette and calm down."

Carol asked the cop, "Do you have a problem with that?"

<u>No</u>, the cop said. <u>You should.</u>

# 129

"I have never seen you like that," Carol's sister said. "I can't believe what you just did. There's not a drill sergeant alive that wouldn't have dropped and given up fifty pushups, the way you were talking. Where did all that come from?"

"No one fucks with Gary," Carol said. "It's not the first time I've had to do that and chances are it won't be the last."

Carol's sister went to stay with Gary.

About five minutes later the head patient advocate came outside and found her.

<u>Mrs. Stern</u>, he said, <u>I promise everything will be fine now.</u>

"And it's in my husband's chart . . . ," Carol started to ask.

<u>He is to be treated as a VIP</u>, the head patient advocate said. <u>Like a king.</u> <u>I put that in his chart.</u>

"I'm sorry you saw that side of me," Carol said. "I'm not normally like that."

<u>Don't apologize</u> the head PA said. <u>I just hope my family members would</u> <u>be the same way.</u>

When Carol entered the ER, it was as if she had walked into a different hospital.

"From the woman at the front desk to the nurses and doctors in the back," Carol said, "every one of them was bending over backwards to make me happy."

When Carol entered Gary's room, the doctor came in behind her.

<u>I have given Mr. Stern some seizure IV medication,</u> he said.

Gary was sleeping.

"But I don't understand," Carol said. "Gary has never needed this medication twice before."

He hasn't had it twice, the doctor said.

"You *did* give it to him the first time," Carol asked. "Right?"

No, the doctor said. I didn't.

"And why not?" Carol asked.

The doctor hesitated for a moment.

Well, he at last said, the cost of one IV is the equivalent to four months of P.O. [pill not liquid] medication.

"Let me get this straight," Carol said. "You didn't treat my husband right the first time because of the cost? Is that what you're telling me?"

It's really not that simple, the doctor said.

"But it is," Carol said. "What you're telling me is you just put money in front of my husband. Let me tell you something. Doctors up in Baltimore tried that, and now look at my husband. They learned the hard way, and it cost them twenty-eight million dollars."

What else can I do for you? the doctor asked.

"I need X-rays of his abdomen," Carol said. "I want to look at them myself, and apparently the PO seizure medicine is not working so I need you to put an order in for liquid medication."

That's not a problem, the doctor said.

When the doctor returned ten minutes later, he said the order was in.

But they had to get it. They didn't have any at this hospital, because they mostly handled beach cases.

"When I have it in my hand," Carol said, "I will then and only then take my husband home."

# 130

---

"While some doctors were on the phones trying to get us out of there," Carol said, "others X-rayed Gary's abdomen."

One doctor started to explain the X-ray to Carol. She stopped him, explaining she had experience—too much experience—reading Gary's X-rays.

Steve from Bear Pharmacy called Carol to let her know he had found some liquid medication. Carol told the doctor, who said he would start the discharge paperwork.

"Not yet," Carol said.

What else do you need us to do?

"I need someone in my husband's room until I get back," Carol said. "My husband will not be discharged until I have his medication in my hand, and I don't want to worry about him while I am gone."

I understand, the doctor said.

"I'll let you know when I have it," Carol said. "Then, you can start the paperwork."

An hour later, Carol was driving Gary home.

# 131

"I needed to get Gary back to his doctors," Carol said, "but we had a lot of problems with Obamacare."

Gary's doctors said they couldn't afford to keep their practices going.

"Some moved to bigger cities," Carol said. "Some closed their offices. Some changed their field of practice."

Gary's doctor McPherson? Closed her office

Gary's GI doctor Kendall? Moved to Pittsburgh.

Carol made appointments after appointments with new doctors, who all said the same thing: Gary's case was too complicated.

"Too complicated?" Carol pointed out she wasn't a doctor, and she had been taking care of Gary.

"I could see Gary giving up," Carol said. "To make matters worse, Gary was becoming tolerant to his regular pain medication dose."

When the checks arrived, Carol wanted to hide them, because she was afraid once Gary knew they had the money to take care of her, he would give up. He would feel that his work was done.

"[S]he wanted me to delay getting it to them," Miller said.

Carol thought when Gary knew she had the check, when he knew she would be taken care of financially, he'd surrender to death.

# 132

Two weeks before Halloween, around 4:30 in the afternoon, Gary and Kenny were in Gary's bedroom.

"I could tell you what Gary and Kenny were doing," Carol said, "but I'm sure you could figure it out."

They had the munchies.

"They always talked about food," Carol said, "but this was over the top."

"I wonder if we can catch crabs in the backyard?" Gary said.

"Sure we can, Pop Pop," Kenny said.

"Do we still have the crab pot?" Gary asked Carol.

Before Carol could answer, Kenny told Gary, "We have everything we need, Pop Pop. Except bait." He asked Carol if she was going food shopping the next day.

"What if I go to the store?" Gary said.

Carol was surprised by Gary's suggestion.

"Babe," Carol said, "if you're feeling up to it."

"I wonder if we'll get a lot of kids on Halloween?" Gary said.

"The kids from the other side of the bridge come over here," Kenny said. "They think the candy's better."

"Babe," Carol asked, "do you want something special this year?"

"I want a bucket full of candy," Gary said. "Half for the Trick-or-Treaters and half for me."

"What about me?" Kenny asked.

"You can have some of the Trick-or-Treaters candy," Gary said.

"I'll make sure Jade comes here first," Kenny said.

"And last." Gary said.

They continued talking about food.

Kenny said, "A new place just opened called Southern Shores Pizza."

Kenny called and ordered a large cheese pizza with extra cheese and light on the sauce.

After hanging up, Kenny said, they would be delivering in about forty minutes. It didn't take that long. Carol had just finished putting out plates when the shop delivered the pizza, which was specially designed for Gary like his TPN: extra cheese and light on the sauce.

Gary and Kenny started eating.

"It's the best pizza I've ever had," Gary said.

"It is really good," Kenny said.

"You're just stoned." Carol said, until she tried a piece.

It was good. Very good.

"Well," Carol said, "one thing you know is crabs and pizza."

"I'm ready to have another piece," Gary said.

"Are you sure, Babe?" Carol asked. "You know what's going to happen."

"This pizza is worth it." Gary said.

Gary was sick for hours after eating the pizza, but the next day he wanted to order again: extra cheese, light on the tomato sauce. At the Southern Shore Pizza Parlor, it became known as a Gary Pizza.

# 133

Gary recovered—and, of course, again got the munchies. But he was in no condition to go to the store. Carol sent Kenny to get a couple of chicken legs. Gary went to the back porch, right outside their bedroom, and watched Kenny put the crab pots in the water.

"Now," Carol said, "I know what you're thinking: It's the wrong time of year. That's what I thought. I was wrong."

Four days later, Gary asked Kenny to check the pots.

"I'm ready for some crabs." Gary said.

Kenny went out into the backyard. Gary stood on the patio outside their bedroom, watching Kenny pull up the farthest pot.

"Something is in here," Kenny said.

"How many?" Gary asked.

"It's a catfish," Kenny said.

"That's no good," Gary said.

"We have two more," Kenny said.

Kenny let the catfish go and started pulling up the second pot.

"There's something in this one, too," Kenny said.

"Another catfish," Gary said.

"Crabs," Kenny said.

"How many?"

"It looks like . . .," Kenny started to say.

"Males?" Gary asked.

"At least five," Kenny said.

"How big?"

Kenny spread his thumb and pinky as far apart as he could and said, "About this big."

"Keepers," Gary said.

Kenny got a bucket into which he put the crabs with ice. Gary went back into his bedroom.

Fifteen minutes later, Kenny came in, carrying the bucket.

"We had fifteen," he said. "But three were females, so I threw them back."

Kenny put on heat under a big pot.

"I'm ready," Gary said.

"For crabs," Carol said. "You're always ready for crabs."

Kenny steamed the crabs. Gary checked on the progress of the crabs half a dozen times.

"It took Gary fifteen minutes to eat six crabs," Carol said. "By the time he finished the sixth, I could hear his stomach going, and, yes, he got sick. He threw up the crabs, but had the biggest smile on his face. Then he ate more crabs."

Carol was watching something everyone had told her would never happen.

Gary was eating crabs.

# 134

Thanksgiving was right around the corner. Peter Angelos's office hired Evelyn Roberts, a nurse and home-care giver, to help Carol take care of Gary.

"She came out to the house a few times," Carol said. "and talked to me on the phone a lot."

Carol liked her.

Carol still was having difficulty finding local doctors for Gary, who wanted everyone to come for the holidays. David and Stacey couldn't make it, but promised to come for Christmas. Kimberly and her husband, Joel, were coming for nine days. Jeanette couldn't make it because she was suffering from shingles. Carol's friend Tanya and her family were coming from Cleveland. Donna couldn't make it. Kenny and Jade would be there. Carol's ex—Robert—was planning to come. Eleven people ended up celebrating with Gary and Carol.

"Gary did it up right," Carol said. "He was so looking forward to the turkey with all the trimmings."

They started preparing ten days before Thanksgiving.

"Gary wanted us to make the dinner together," Carol said. "Unfortunately, Gary was so over-stimulated that he had a bad time the Wednesday night before the big day. Thursday morning, he was in bad shape."

Carol was running back and forth between the bedroom and the kitchen. Kimberly and Joel helped in the kitchen. Tanya's baby girl was on TPN; she knew about central lines, so she helped Carol with Gary.

When they sat down for dinner, the head of the table—Gary's chair—was empty.

"Gary," Carol said, "didn't eat that day. But the next day, he was all about the pies."

It was a warm November. Carol settled Gary on the back porch.

Everyone was swimming in the pool or on the dock fishing. Gary and Carol sat for hours watching. At one point, Carol thought Gary had gone into a trance.

"Are you okay, Babe?" Carol asked.

Gary came out of his trance.

"Huh?" Gary said. "Were you saying something?"

"Yes, Babe. Are you all right?"

"I was thinking about something."

"What were you thinking about?"

"About how you're missing out on everything."

"What are you talking about?"

"You should be out there with everyone having fun, not sitting here with me."

"Babe, I'm right where I want to be, right next to you."

Kenny and Joel were catching fish after fish.

"Look, Pop Pop," Kenny called, holding up a fish. "It's a big one."

"Look, Pop Pop," Jade called. "Look what I can do."

Jade cannonballed into the pool.

"My fish was bigger," Joel called, "wasn't it, Paw Paw?" (Not Pop Pop. Joel had his own nickname for Gary.)

Kimberly came over to them and asked, "Can I get you anything, Gary?"

No nickname.

"I'm good," Gary said.

And he was. He was having fun watching all of them.

"You know" Kimberly said, "I caught the biggest fish with my net."

"Ya," Gary said, "I saw that."

Nadilla called out, "Paw Paw, Paw Paw, watch me."

"Okay, Nadilla, I'm watching."

Nadilla jumped into the pool.

"Did you see, Paw Paw? Did you see?"

"Yes, Nadilla. That's was really good. But be careful."

"I will Paw Paw," Nadilla said, "I will."

Princess and Zenny were in the backyard, playing with the ball. Butchy lay by Gary's feet.

Kenny pulled the crab pods up one by one, glancing over at Gary.

"No crabs today, Pop Pop," Kenny said.

"That's all right," Gary called back. "We have turkey."

Carol took Gary's hand.

"You see, Babe," Carol said, "everyone is calling out for you. Everyone wants you to be a part of everything, and I'm right where I want to be."

Gary smiled.

"I love you, Baby Doll," Gary said.

"I love you, too, Babe," Carol said.

At last, life seemed back to normal.

# 135

---

Too soon, suitcases and duffels were packed in various cars. Everyone was going home.

Thanksgiving was over. Even the leftovers were over.

"After everyone went home, Gary and I needed to get back to some peace, which was not easy," Carol said. "I wanted to take care of Gary, and Gary wanted to focus on Christmas. And getting out of pain."

Equinox was not available in Carol and Gary's new area, and there were some problems with the new pharmacy that was supplying Gary with TPN and other medications, including his IV pain killer.

"We had been using this company for a little over a year with all types of problems, such as deliveries being late, deliveries not sent out, getting someone else's delivery, missing things in the delivery," Carol said. "But my biggest problem with them was that I didn't have to sign for Gary's pain medication."

The UPS driver would leave the packages on the driveway.

"In the smaller house it wasn't that bad because it was a smaller town and we could hear the driver pull up," Carol said. But Duck Woods was larger. The UPS drivers would leave the medications halfway down the driveway.

"This was a big problem for more than one reason," Carol said.

Another list.

1.  Gary's TPN had to be kept between 36° to 45°F.
2.  Gary's pain medication was sitting in the driveway, unattended until someone noticed it. Anyone could to come by and take it.

Carol repeatedly, unsuccessfully, asked the new pharmacy to make sure the driver had someone sign for the packages.

"I didn't understand why Gary's pain medication was running out early," Carol said. So Carol and Miss Janet started weighing the pain-killer cartridges. The first few times the weight was off. But after Carol started tracking the pain killers—and telling the sender that she was weighing the drugs—the cartridges started to weigh the right amount.

But the company called Gary's pain management doctor and accused Carol of selling the drugs or using them herself.

Carol told the doctor that he could test her anytime and that they didn't need the money.

"I just needed to make Gary comfortable," Carol said. "The doctor didn't want to hear it. He dropped Gary as a patient."

Carol had sixty days to find a new doctor.

*What the hell is going on,* Carol wondered, *and what do I do now? This is bullshit.*

"I don't care what they think of me," Carol said, "but I can't let Gary down."

He needed his TPN, he needed his pain killers.

"If these people knew me," Carol said, "they would know better."

*Okay,* Carol said to herself. *What do I do?*

Pray.

"But," Carol said, "sometimes Satan gets in the way."

Miss Janet kept Gary's spirits up with singing and talking about when she worked with Mother Teresa, and the work she was doing at a Women's Battered Shelter.

Not all were cheerful topics, but all were compelling. And distracting.

Gary was interested in her work at the Women's Battered Shelter, because he knew of Carol's history of being assaulted.

He felt it was important to help the shelter out. He gave them a new dishwasher, and a refrigerator.

# 136

Chad arrived with a random ham.

"A <u>random</u> ham." Carol laughed.

Gary gave it to the Battered Women's Shelter.

The shelter named a fund Gary started after him.

"Gary wanted it named after me," Carol said. "I wanted it named after him."

It was going to be called "The Gary and Carol Birthday Fund."

"I said no," Carol said. "It's The Gary Stern Birthday Fund."

The donation helped support advocates, because —Carol said—"in order for people to get better, they need strong advocates. What they need to know is, when you have someone that you love and they're sick and they get angry or they seem impossible or they say things that are really hurtful, you have to realize they're not talking to you. Chances are that they're scared, or they're yelling at death. Like Gary."

Advocates can also help in hospitals with something as simple as making sure every hospital room has a chair that can fold down into a bed if someone wants to spend the night with a loved one.

"You wouldn't believe some of the things I've slept on," Carol said. "Window sills. Straight-back chairs."

She still has back pain from some of the odd places where she had to sleep.

# 137

Gary had enough TPN, medication, and painkillers to last until after Christmas.

"He was so looking forward to it," Carol said, "I tried to focus on Christmas."

Gary told Carol he wanted everybody here for Christmas.

"Kelly decorated the house for me, right, because everybody was coming. She even wrapped presents. And Gary was telling me it was going to be his very last Christmas."

"It was a tragic moment," Carol said. "It was also a triumphant moment."

Anyone can die at any moment.

"A cop could shoot me by mistake," Carol said. "Or I could get trampled by a herd of pygmy *elephants* because the circus is in town . . ."

"You never know," David said.

"But," Carol said about Gary, "here's a guy who confronted his death, and he was able to say, 'I know this is my last Christmas, and that's okay, because I'm going to make it a good Christmas.'"

Carol had confirmed Christmas with everyone who was coming. Gary was elated. Kimberly and Nadilla would be getting in ten days before the holiday. Joel was coming four days before. David, Stacey, and Shannon, their daughter, were driving down five days before.

Gary was proud of Shannon, who had become a lawyer like her grandfather Sonny. Even though Taylor, David and Stacey's other daughter, a fourth-grade school teacher, couldn't come because she was in India, "It was a happy time for us," Carol said.

Kenny draped lights over the front of the house. More important, he made sure the back of the house looked magical. He put lights around the back porch, around the pool, around the dock, and in their tree.

"Gary would be spending most of his time in our bedroom," Carol said.

From there, Gary had a view of the decorations in the back.

It was unseasonably warm two days before Kimberly and Nadilla were due to fly in. About 8:30 at night, Carol and Gary were in the bedroom, Gary in his favorite chair and Carol on the bed when they heard music coming from the backyard. Carol got up and looked out back, but didn't see anything unusual.

The music got louder.

"Turn the sound down." Gary assumed the music was coming from a TV in another room.

Carol did, too.

At first.

The music got louder.

"Is that Christmas music?" Gary asked.

"I think it is," Carol said.

She opened the sliding glass door to the back porch. Gary walked over to her.

"Where is it coming from?" he asked.

"I have no idea," Carol said.

"Is that 'Silent Night'?"

"Yes," Carol said, "it is."

"Let's go out back," Gary said.

Carol helped Gary shrug on his bathrobe.

"We then stepped out onto the porch," Carol said.

The music was very loud.

Gary pointed to the canal behind their house.

"Baby doll," he said, "look over there."

"Where?"

"In the water."

Christmas lights were approaching.

It was a boat parade. Eight or nine boats were all lit up. Gary and Carol heard the people on the boat singing along with the music. As each boat went by people called out Christmas greetings.

Gary took Carol's hand. With his free hand, he waved.

"Merry Christmas to you, too" Gary called.

At that moment, Carol felt Gary reentering normal life.

As the last boat passed, Gary squeezed Carol's hand.

"Merry Christmas, Baby Doll," he said.

"Merry Christmas, Babe," Carol said.

"This is going to be our best Christmas ever," Gary said.

"With many more to come," Carol said.

"Looking back at it now," Carol said, "Gary knew it was going to be his last because he squeezed my hand a little more and said: "I love you, Baby Doll, and I will always be with you."

# 138

David took Gary shopping.

"He was like a kid in Wal-Mart," David said. "He was going crazy."

"I'm going to get Gary a ball for Christmas," Nadilla said, remembering what Gary had told her about why his belly was distended, "because you know what he does with balls."

"It is the triumph that comes out of suffering," Carol said. "That leads to a kind of understanding about the human condition, which you can share with others, who are not going to be blindsided by it as you originally were. You are a witness. You can give testimony to the fact that, when the hammer comes down, you do what you can, but you don't let it get you down."

"Carol never showed Gary she was repelled by his condition," David said. "She never let him see her cry. She was indomitable, because that's what Gary needed, and Gary was being indomitable, because that was what Carol needed."

"Gary may have been somewhat ready to go," said Kelly, "but Carol, absolutely not. At no time, no way, no how."

Some of the other family members might have been half accepting Gary's death, but not Carol.

Carol confirmed the guest list: David, Stacey, Shannon, Kimberly, Joel, Nadilla, Kenny, Jade, Jade's sister Amber, Jade's mom, her step dad, and even Carol's ex, Robert. Everyone important to Gary was coming.

Kelly helped Carol get the house ready.

By the time Kimberly and Nadilla flew in from California, everything was ready except for the tree.

"Gary and I were so excited to see them," Carol said. "We hadn't spent the holidays with Kimberly in years and had never spent the Christmas holidays with Nadilla, who was five years old (a good age for kids at Christmas)."

It was the first Christmas Gary and Carol would have their kids and their grandkids and David and Stacey and Shannon.

"Oh," Carol said, "oh, and, of course, my ex-Robert."

A couple of days after Kimberly and Nadilla got in, it was time to go pick out a tree, so Kimberly and Kenny went with the girls (Jade, Nadilla), who were so excited when they got back home, all they wanted to do was tell (Pop Pop, Paw Paw) about the tree they both ran into his bedroom.

"He was in pain," David said, "but he didn't want to show it."

# 139

At 4:30 on Christmas Eve, Nadilla came into Gary's bedroom.

"Ha, little girl," Gary said, "are you ready for Santa?"

"Not yet, Paw Paw," Nadilla said. "I haven't had dinner, my shower, brushed my teeth, and we need to put out cookies for Santa and his reindeer."

"His reindeer? Do they eat cookies?"

"No, Paw Paw, they eat oranges and carrots."

"Do we have any oranges and carrots, Nana?" Gary asked Carol.

"We have carrots," Carol said, "but no oranges."

"Nana," Nadilla told Carol, "we need oranges."

"But we have carrots," Carol said.

"The reindeer get tired of just carrots," Nadilla said.

"How about some bananas?" Gary asked Nadilla.

"That's silly, Paw Paw." Nadilla said.

"Okay," Gary told Carol, "you heard her. We need oranges."

Gary called out to Joel.

"Can you come in here for a minute?"

Joel came into the bedroom.

"What's up," he asked.

"Can you go to the store for me and get some oranges?" Gary asked.

"Some oranges?" Joel asked.

"Daddy," Nadilla said, "we need them for the reindeer."

"But we have carrots," Joel said.

The reindeer are tired of carrots," Gary said.

"It's after four," Joel said. "The stores are all closed, but I'll go look."

Joel went to three stores. They were all closed. At a 7/11, he found oranges.

A few hours later, Carol and Nadilla put out the cookies, milk, carrots, and oranges.

"Paw Paw," Nadilla called, "come look."

Gary looked and approved.

Kimberly took Nadilla to bed and was going to come back down two hours later to take care of Santa's presents, but instead Joel came downstairs and told them Kimberly was sick.

Carol started Gary's TPN, and he had fallen asleep. Shannon and David had gone to bed, so it was up to Stacey, Joel, and Carol to be Santa.

Carol and Stacey didn't finish wrapping presents and stuffing stockings until four in the morning.

"Stacey and I had so much fun we laughed all night," Carol said. "It's really funny watching a Jewish girl play Santa."

# 140

Christmas morning, Carol got up early. By seven, everyone—except for Kimberly, who was sick—was awake. Kenny and Jade were still at their house. Joel kept Nadilla upstairs for about an hour, so Carol (feeling like a drill sergeant) could deploy the rest of the family organizing holiday surprises.

Kimberly managed to come downstairs. Joel and Nadilla also came down. They all gathered in the living room. Including Gary.

"Nadilla was so excited," Carol said.

Instead of running to her presents, Nadilla went to the stockings hanging along the fireplace mantel, where, starting at the left-hand side, she unhooked Gary's stocking and carried it to Gary.

"Here, Paw Paw," she said. "Don't look yet."

"Why not," Gary teased her, "it's mine, right?"

"It's only fair," Nadilla said, "if you wait for everyone."

"That's a great idea," Gary said.

"I know," Nadilla said. "I thought of it myself."

Nadilla handed out stockings to Carol, Kimberly, Joel, and Robert, to everyone who was there. She looked around, running back and forth, up and down, and turning around.

"Nadilla," Joel asked, "what are you doing?"

"I'm looking for stockings," Nadilla said.

"You handed out all the stockings," Joel said. "Now, you get yours."

"No, Daddy," Nadilla said. "I need three more."

Everyone exchanged glances.

"Oh," Gary said. "For the dogs."

"No, Paw Paw." Nadilla pointed to David, Stacey, and Shannon, who were gathered at the bar.

"There's . . ." Nadilla hesitated.

"You can probably figure out what we are all thinking," Carol said. David, Stacey, and Shannon celebrated Hanukah not Christmas. "How do we tell a five-year-old about Judaism?"

"We left our stockings at home," Stacey said, "so Santa could go to our house."

"Okay, then," Nadilla said, "everyone can look inside their stocking now."

Kimberly and Joel let Nadilla open their presents from Santa. They'd open the rest of the presents when Kenny and Jade arrived.

"The plan was, Kenny and Jade would be here at about one," Carol said. "I would start dinner, then we'd open the rest of the presents. But, you know what they say about the best laid plans."

Carol knew something was going to go wrong.

"And it did," Carol said. "Kimberly needed to lay back down. Then, five minutes after Kenny got here, Jade needed to lay down, sick as Kimberly. Then, Kenny, then Robert, also feeling sick, needed to go home. The family was dropping like flies."

To protect Gary, Carol secluded him in their bedroom room and started spraying Lysol all over the house.

"We managed to open all the presents except for Jade's, who also was sick," Carol said. "God love her, she tried to keep the holiday spirits up, but she was too sick."

Kenny took her to his house to recover.

David and Stacey didn't get sick but they decided to go back to Baltimore a little earlier then planed.

By seven that night, Nadilla started getting sick.

"For the next week," Carol said, "they all had the flu."

Gary and Carol escaped, but Carol wouldn't let Gary out of the bedroom, and she wouldn't let anyone in.

"Needless to say, I didn't make a Christmas dinner that year." Carol confessed. "But I did make a lot of chicken soup.

# 141

___

For the next few days after Christmas, Carol was worried that Gary was going to get the flu, which could be dangerous since Gary's immune system was compromised. Kimberly was still sick. Nadilla was running a 102.6 temperature and needed antibiotics. Joel was sick, but it didn't stop him from taking care of Kimberly and Nadilla. Kenny was sick and taking care of Jade.

Five days after Christmas, Gary vitals were bad. His blood pressure was low, his heart rate was high. His temperature was low, and his anger was high.

All signs that Gary was septic.

Carol took Gary to the ER. The nurses stayed in the room with Gary while Carol was at the nurses' station with a doctor.

One of the nurses came out of Gary's room and told the doctor that Gary wouldn't let her start a IV line.

"We have to start new line," the doctor said. "His current central line is infected. If we don't start a new line, he will die within hours."

Carol said, "I'll take care of it."

To the nurse, she said, "Come with me."

The nurse hesitated until the doctor told her to go with Carol. In Gary's room, Gary said to Carol, "Tell her not to stick me, please." Everything was supposed to be back to normal. Christmas had been normal—not what

Gary had been expecting, but not bad—and now here he was back in a hospital with one of the same old problems.

Carol explained that the nurse had to put a new line in.

"I'm tired," Gary said.

"Listen to me," Carol said, "your central line is infected. If she doesn't put a new line in, you're going to die. Are you ready to die?"

"No, no," Gary said.

"Okay, good," Carol said. "I don't want you to die."

After the nurse put in a peripheral line, the doctor came into the room and said that Gary was being transferred to a hospital in Virginia, to their ICU. The doctors in the ICU wanted to put in yet another new central line. Gary begged them to save the one he had.

"Gary's had been in for the last year and a half," Carol said. "The doctors would tell us, Gary had so much scar tissue that this was going to be Gary's last central line. They all also said Gary only had days to live."

# 142

On every New Year's Eve, even during the past four years when Gary was in hospitals, Gary and Carol managed to watch the ball drop in Times Square on television and kiss at midnight. This year was no different. And it felt to both Gary and Carol that this was the most important New Year's ever. Unspoken was the question: Would it be their last New Year's?

Gary was in the ICU, sitting up in his bed. Carol sat in a chair next to him. They held hands.

"As the ball dropped, I looked over at Gary to say Happy New Year," Carol said. "And Gary was sound asleep. He'd had such a hard couple of days, I didn't have the heart to wake him."

At midnight, Carol kissed his hand and whispered, "Happy New Year's, my darling. I love you."

# 143

On January 3, Gary got his new central line.

They got home from the hospital on January 7 in a good mood. It looked like things were finally going to be okay. The first thing Gary wanted to do after saying hi to the kids and grandkids was to eat Donna's Momma Donna pie.

He sang "I'm gonna eat Momma Donna pie" at least ten times.

Carol finally told Gary about the check, which was in the safe.

"Carol told me she was worried," David said, "that when all the money was there—if Gary knew—he was going to let go."

Carol gave Gary's Glock to David. She was afraid she might use it. On herself.

# 144

February 9, 2016.

A woman came to Gary and Carol's door. She said she was from Adult Family Services.

"I was called by someone," the Adult Family Services rep said. "I can't tell you who, but I was told to come check on a Mr. Stern. Is he here?"

"Yes," Carol said. "I'm his wife."

Instead of inviting the AFS rep in, because Carol didn't want Gary to overhear what Carol suspected would be an unpleasant conversation, Carol stepped outside to talk to her.

"I don't need to know how or why someone called you," Carol said, "but thank you for coming."

"Can we go inside?" the AFS rep asked.

"Yes," Carol said, "absolutely, but first I need to tell you a few things."

"Okay," the AFS rep said. "What is it?"

"First and foremost," Carol said, "I cannot let anyone get my husband upset. You can ask me anything you would like and come by anytime, but please don't let on to my husband that someone called you about me. When he gets upset, my husband is prone to having seizures."

Since Gary and Carol had recently moved to Dare County, the AFS rep could make it sound like normal practice to visit anyone new to the area who was on palliative care.

That way, Carol explained, "My husband would be okay about anything you ask."

They went inside the house. Carol asked her to stay in the living room for just a minute so she could make sure Gary was dressed and to let him know someone was here to see them.

Carol kept Gary's bedroom door open so the AFS rep could hear their conversation.

"I didn't want her to think I had anything to hide," Carol said.

After checking on Gary, Carol asked the AFS rep to come into the bedroom. Carol made the introductions.

"Babe," Carol said to Gary, "she is from Dare County. She just stopped by to see how we are settling into the house."

"We're doing all right," Gary said.

"Is there anything we can do?" The AFS rep asked.

"My wife takes care of everything we need," Gary said. "She's my angel."

"That's great to hear," the AFS rep said.

"I'm going to let you talk for a minute," Carol said, "and I will be right back."

"Where are you going?" Gary asked.

"I need to go to the restroom," Carol said.

"Okay, Baby Doll," Gary said.

Carol left them alone.

"I didn't need to go to the restroom," Carol said, "but I felt it was important for her to talk to Gary alone. I had nothing to hide."

Carol planned to give them ten minutes, but after five minutes the AFS rep came into the living room, where Carol was waiting.

Carol walked her outside, where the AFS rep said, "Thank you for giving me some time alone with your husband."

"Thank you for coming out," Carol said, "and especially for not upsetting my husband."

"I can tell that you're taking excellent care of your husband," the AFS rep said. "The state requires that we make three visits to the home."

"Stop by anytime day or night," Carol said. "If I'm not here, the nurse will be here. I don't leave Gary alone. Too many things can go wrong."

# 145

A few days later, Carol was on the front porch waiting for Gary's medication to show up, making sure no one stole the painkillers, when the AFS rep arrived for the second visit.

"Hello, again," she said. "How is everything going today?"

"Gary seems to be having a good day," Carol said. "Right now he's sleeping, but I can hear him if he needs me. I have a room monitor on him."

They sat down outside on two folding chairs.

"I understand you have a job to do," Carol said, "and I don't have a problem with you stopping by. However, I can't go inside right now because I'm waiting for Gary's medication."

"You have to wait for it outside?"

Carol was explaining the situation, when Miss Janet drove up. Carol introduced them and explained that the AFS rep was there to see how Gary is doing.

"I don't take care of Gary," Miss Janet said.

She helped Carol take care of Gary.

Carol went inside to see if Gary was still sleeping and to give them time to talk alone. When Carol went back outside, she overheard Miss Janet saying, "I've been a RN for more than thirty years. I have an impeccable reputation in the community with hospice and palliative care. Mr. Stern is a very sick man; and, if it wasn't for Mrs. Stern, he would have died many years ago. She is by far one of the best caregivers I've seen. I know about these accusations, of Carol's drug use and mistreatment of Gary, and I'm here to say they are not true."

Miss Janet went inside, passing Carol who sat down next to the AFS rep.

"Gary is still sleeping," Carol said. "Can you wait a little bit for him to wake up? I don't let anyone disturb his sleep."

Carol was direct.

"If you have been called out here because of the accusations about me selling or taking my husband's medication, I will tell you the same thing I've told others. If anyone has seen what I've seen my husband go through, they would know how ridiculous the accusations would be. I don't know how anyone could take medication from someone in that much pain, and there is no way in hell I would let that happen to my husband."

At which point the UPS driver pulled up.

"Well, look at that," Carol said. "Now, watch. The driver will take two boxes off his truck and put them halfway down the driveway without me signing for them."

A week's worth of Gary's IV Dilaudid were in one of the boxes.

"So," Carol said, "we sat there" watching the driver do just what Carol had predicted.

Carol excused herself.

"Miss Janet and I need to bring the boxes in," Carol said, "put the TPN in the refrigerator, and we need to weigh the Dilaudid cartridges because they've been weighing light. You can come in and watch us if you would like."

"I've seen enough," the AFS rep said. "I do have to come out one more time even though I don't feel it's necessary. I don't see any truth to the accusations."

## 146

After Adult Family Services was sicced on Carol, she lost her patience with the new pharmacy that had been supplying Gary's drugs.

"I didn't have the time or the energy to put up with it," Carol said. "I needed and only wanted to focus on what was important. On Gary."

She called her old friend, Mason from Equinox in Baltimore, who told Carol that Equinox had opened an office in North Carolina.

"That was music to my ears," Carol said. "It took me all of an hour to have everything moved back to Equinox."

Mason FedEx'ed everything overnight to them.

"So," Mason said, "it was a little bit more work from a logistical stand-point, but we continued to take care of them . . . [Gary] had pain control issues and he was going to require IV pain medicine, either Morphine or Dilaudid . . ."

Mason understood what Gary and Carol were going through was more than a medical or legal story. It was a love story.

# 147

They didn't know it, but Gary had three weeks to live.

Gary was still having bad days. He was in and out of the hospital for brief periods. The longest stay was overnight for IV antibiotics, because it could take twenty-four hours to get new antibiotics delivered to the house. Gary couldn't wait.

Finally, Carol felt everything going right.

"We started talking about the future," Carol said, "something we hadn't done in a very, very long time."

They wanted to build a house with their bedroom on the top floor and a big skylight so they could lie in bed and look up at the stars. And a balcony that overlooked the ocean. And a bedroom for the dogs. And a room for Kenny, Kimberly, and Joel, and the grandkids.

"Oh, yes," Carol said, "and a bedroom for David and Stacey."

They made plans to go West. Gary wanted to stop in Las Vegas to play blackjack.

"We were going to spend time with his childhood friend, Steven Levi," Carol said, "and spend time with Kimberly, Joel, and, of course, Nadilla."

Carol checked on how to get Butchy papers to be a service dog, so he could go with them.

They talked about visiting Baltimore for an O's game and a Ravens game.

"It had been such a long time coming," Carol said. "We were talking about our future together, and it was wonderful."

Gary kept saying, "It's going to be great, Baby Doll. I'm going to take care of you in every way."

Since Gary had gotten sick, their love life was like Gary's passion for food—they talked about what they would do once Gary got well.

"I love you, Baby Doll," Gary said.

# 148

Gary's perception of time was gone.

"As soon as I would walk out of the room to do something," Carol said, "Gary called me back. He was scared that something would happen. He was having a lot of seizures. He wanted to make sure that I was there. Even if I was asleep, if I was in the bedroom, he was okay. Even if David was taking care of him, or Kenny was taking care of him, or Stacey, he was okay, so long as I was there."

Gary was losing weight. Not good.

"Kenny took us to Virginia to see Dr. Gaglione," Carol said.

Kenny always took them, because Carol was always worried about Gary having seizures.

"We were on our way back home," Carol said. "It was a good visit. Gary really liked this doctor."

They stopped to get something to eat, a turkey sandwich for Carol. When she took the first bite, "half of my top teeth fell out."

"I'm not sure who was more upset about it," Carol said, "me or Gary."

For days Gary hounded Carol about going to the dentist.

"I couldn't help but think it was more important for Gary to go to the dentist," Carol said.

The day before Gary went into the hospital for the last time, they promised each other to go to the dentist together."

"It was the first promise I couldn't keep with Gary," Carol said. "And the last."

# 149

Friday, March 4, 2016.

Gary was having a good day. Almost back to his old self.    .

"He was even talking about getting frisky," Carol said.

But Carol couldn't shake a feeling of something bad impending, which she hid from Gary.

"I had a feeling he knew what I was feeling," Carol said. "He always knew."

Carol couldn't sleep. She sat watching Gary sleeping.

"I haven't told anyone this next part, not even David or Kenny," Carol said. "If only had I talked to Gary sooner."

The next afternoon, Gary came from the bathroom, sat in his chair, and, eyes getting bigger, grabbed his chest as if he was having a heart attack. Carol caught him.

"Are you all right?" she asked.

"Wow," Gary said. "I'm okay now. Boy, I never want to feel that way ever again."

"We need to go to the hospital and get that checked out," Carol said.

"No," Gary said. "I'm okay now."

"I'm calling the doctor," Carol said.

"No, I'm good."

"I'm going to check your blood pressure."

"Stop fussing over me."

"Gary, we are going to the hospital, or I'm taking your blood pressure."

"Take my blood pressure, damn it."

Gary had a little tachycardia, but his blood pressure seemed fine.

Carol's dread increased. For the next three days, she didn't sleep for more than twenty minutes.

Kenny had been staying at his place. Carol had no in-house back-up.

On Tuesday morning, Carol drifted off about eight-thirty. Kelly was due to arrive at nine.

Carol woke up at nine-fifteen. Gary was standing next to his chair, eating a peanut butter and jelly sandwich.

"Morning, Baby Doll," Gary said. "Kelly is here."

"Good morning, sweetheart," Carol said. "Do you need your medicine?"

His painkiller.

"I'm okay," Gary said, "until you get your coffee."

"I'll be back in five minutes." Carol said.

Carol went into the kitchen. Kelly had made the coffee. Carol poured a cup and sat at the bar with Kelly. For a minute or two they chatted, when Butchy started crying—not a bark or a whine, a cry.

"It was like Butchy telling me it was time," Carol said.

Carol told Kelly, "Something's wrong with Gary."

She ran into the bedroom.

"I . . . thought she was jumping the gun," Kelly said, "because we would have good days and bad days. We had days where Gary was very upbeat, and days where he was like, 'All the fucking money in the world can't make this go away . . .' That was . . . how he said it . . . It didn't matter what the end judgement was . . . There was no dollar amount that could fix what had happened to him . . . Some days . . . you could tell he was down about the hand that had been dealt him, because this is a man in the prime of his life . . ."

He had been running a fever, not high—hundred, a hundred and one, maybe a hundred and two—but that didn't seem abnormal to Kelly.

"It wasn't anything that like made me feel . . . we had to . . . take him to the hospital or anything."

"Call 911," Carol told Kelly. "Do it now."

"Babe," Carol said to Gary, "you have to go to the hospital."

Usually, Gary would say, "No, I'm fine," but this time he looked Carol in the eyes and said, "It's time to let me go, Baby Doll."

# 150

Carol sat Gary in his chair.

Kelly put Zenny and Princess in the bathroom and shut the door. She went outside to wait for the ambulance.

Normally, Carol would be getting everything ready to take to the hospital. Not this time.

She sat on the floor next to Gary, who held her hand.

"It's okay," Gary said. "I'm ready for this. I'm going to be all right now, Baby Doll, and so are you. You know you're my angel."

"I didn't know then," Carol said, "but that was the last conversation we had. It was the last time I saw Gary's beautiful brown eyes. If only I knew . . ."

"I had been here for two months with Carol," Kelly said, "and we had formed a friendship . . . You can't help but love people when you take care of them . . ."

Even though she was hired to take care of Gary, she felt as if she had to take care of Carol, too, "because here was this woman who had just run herself into the ground taking care of her husband. And I couldn't help but love . . . her."

Twenty minutes later or so, when the EMTs arrived, Kelly thought "they were being rough with Gary."

Gary was so afraid that Kelly worried they would hurt him.

"Freeze," Kelly said. "This is my patient . . . We're going to regroup here, because this man is very ill, and you all are being too rough."

She admitted, "I had to be a bitch."

Carol, getting dressed in the bathroom, heard Kelly.

"I wanted them to treat Gary gently," Kelly said.

And, after she bawled them out, they did.

"Every time we called 911, Gary would fight," Carol said. "He didn't fight that day."

# 151

In the ambulance, Gary was intubated, so his last words remained, "I'm ready to go."

The EMS took Gary to the Outer Banks Hospital. From there, he was helicoptered to Princess Anne's Hospital in [Norfolk,] Virginia.

Kelly thought it was "weird" that they never got "a signal" from Gary, which often happens.

It "caught me off . . . guard," Kelly said. "I really did not think he was going to pass away anytime soon. I didn't . . . Carol was like nurse du jour, and I thought this could go on for years."

"We really got to the point where we didn't think it was ever going to happen," Miss Janet said.

He had beaten the odds for so long.

"He was enjoying life," Miss Janet said.

Enjoying his lamb chops and the Stooges and the crabs from O'Neal's Seafood Harvest.

Men "can be the worst patients," Kelly said.

But Gary "appreciated good service . . ." Miss Janet said, "and he was very loyal."

When "you're resigned to being at home," Kelly said, "you look for . . . certain people" who make up part of your reduced world—like," Miss Janet said, "the pizza guy."

"The pizza guy was important," Miss Janet said.

Gary—Miss Janet said—he "bore [his condition] with grace and dignity and much courage."

She thought that "with hospice patients, it's all about hope, even if that hope entails having a pain-free death . . . "

And Carol "was able to instantly separate the wheat from the chaff . . . She gets right down to the nitty-gritty."

Miss Janet continued, "I'm going to say something crude, but I guess it's okay . . . Carol had the balls to be an extraordinarily efficient advocate."

Doctors can be competitive. An ER doctor kept ignoring a patient's complaints about constipation. He apologized. He knew he wasn't being attentive. He explained, when he was with other doctors, one might say, "I just did a brain transplant," and all the other doctors go, "Oh, how wonderful, how wonderful." Another doctor might say, "Well, I just transplanted a brain and every organ in some guy's body." The other doctors would say, "How wonderful." A third doctor might say, "I just transplanted a whole personality." The other doctors say, "Oh, how fantastic." And all I could say is, "I helped a guy take a shit . . ."

"I wasn't paying attention to you," the doctor told the patient, "because you're not interesting enough."

"Eighty percent of a hospital staff is wonderful," Carol said. "Fifteen percent are burned out, 5 percent . . .they're in the wrong business."

Carol was worried Gary was going to give up: that once he got a verdict and he knew he was vindicated, and he knew there was money to take care of Carol, there was nothing left to fight for.

"He stopped fighting because his fight was over," Carol said. "He had won."

"After my pop passed, Gary was talking about us being put to rest in West Virginia next to mom and pop, talking and looking at coffins," Carol said.

Gary was shopping for a coffin online, and, because the internet never forgets a search, Carol still gets calls about Gary, inquiring about life insurance.

"While David was visiting, Gary told him where he wanted to be put to rest," Carol said.

"It was not an easy time."

# 152

Kimberly was in California, when Donna called and said, "He's gonna die."

Of course, Kimberly knew who "he" was.

"That's what's gonna happen right now," her cousin said. "Like, it's done."

"I'm on my way out," Kimberly said.

When Kimberly arrived on the East Coast, "everybody was at a stand-still. His sister-in-law and his brother, you could see it on their faces immediately, they didn't know what to do."

They were in shock.

"They didn't know what they were doing," Kimberly said. "My brother didn't know what to do. They had worked so hard while he was alive, and, as soon as he died, they were done. They were burnt."

At the hospital, Gary was maxed out on all medications. He went back on a respirator. Carol asked the doctors what Gary's blood gasses were. When she heard, she knew Gary was in trouble.

"When he'd come close before," Carol said, she was always sure Gary "would come out of it."

But now, Carol said, "I knew he couldn't survive."

At the Sentara Hospital in Virginia, when Carol decided she had to disconnect all life-support from Gary, she arranged to have his family there. Gary was in the ICU.

"The doctor told me Gary had water on his heart and water in his lungs," Carol said, "and there was no coming back."

"Is he brain dead?" Carol asked.

Not yet, the doctor said.

"So, my husband can hear me?" Carol asked.

Yes, the doctor said.

"If I had kept him on life support," Carol said, "there was so much water on his heart that he would have had a massive heart attack. He would have died in pain. He went through so much, for so long, I wasn't going to let him go out that way."

Carol always slept with her glasses on, "because"—Carol said—"I didn't have the luxury of waking up and trying to find my glasses."

When Gary needed her, she jumped up.

"And that's where God, angels, whoever it was, always, or Butchy, always woke me up to let me know that something was about to happen to Gary," Carol said. "I was always up right before something severe happened to Gary. And I, I don't know why, but it's like we were connected. The night before Gary passed away, I heard Gary, he was intubated, he was on life support, and I heard Gary say, "Come change me, I'm wet." Now, I was asleep, and I heard that. All right? And it was about the same time that it always was, and I had done this in ICU units before, and I've done it in hospitals before. I would get up and I would go straight to Gary, and I would start just changing him, just doing whatever needed to be done, and I always knew what it was. I woke up that night and it was like Gary was inside my head telling me that he was wet, and cold. And I went over to him and I felt him, and he was wet, he had had an accident, so I started cleaning him up. The nurse came in and started yelling at me because I was touching Gary, and I was doing things that I wasn't supposed to do. It was a different hospital" (Sentara Princess Anne Hospital in Virginia Beach, Virginia). "They didn't know me yet."

Carol explained that Gary woke her up. The nurse looked at Gary.

He can't talk, the nurse said.

"He can talk to me," Carol said. "He woke me up."

The nurse asked what she was doing.

"He's wet," Carol said. "He needs to be changed, he needs to be cleaned up and changed."

I'll do it, the nurse said.

"Okay," Carol said, "fine."

She kissed Gary on the hand.

"The nurse is going to change you," Carol told Gary.

The next morning, when Carol woke up, two people hovered over her, telling her there had been a problem the night before, "and that I was doing stuff to Gary that I wasn't supposed to do," Carol said. "And I said, 'No, I was doing stuff to Gary that I've always done.'"

"We don't know why you would do that," the doctors said.

"No one ever does," Carol said, "but I do it."

They weren't listening to Carol, so she called Donna, who came.

"You don't understand what this woman and this man have been through," Donna said. "You need to go look at their file."

"I don't know what else Donna said," Carol said, "but I got an apology, and I said, 'Don't worry about it, we understand.'"

When David and Stacey and other family members arrived, Carol told the nurse, "My husband's going to pass away."

"Yes," she said.

"I will be the one that washes him off and gets him ready after he passes away," Carol told her.

"I have to [check with] the charge nurse on that," she says. "We've never had anyone ask that. Why are you asking?"

"I've been bathing my husband ever since he got sick," Carol said. "I've been changing fistula bags, I've been changing central lines, I keep his labs, I can tell you every lab he's got. This is the last bath that he's going to get, and you're going to deprive me of that?"

"Are you aware of what you're going to see?" she asked.

"Yeah," Carol said. "I'm going to see my husband have a bath, without pain. I don't care about his movements. I've cleaned up his movements for years. I know what's going to happen. I'm cleaning him up."

Carol didn't know if Gary heard her last words to him.

"Gary," she said, "with all the love in your heart, please let me know you're okay."

Gary didn't squeeze Carol's hand, but a tear was running down his cheek.

"You know I love you," Carol said. "And I know you can hear me. I will be with you again, but this you have to do on your own. And you're not going to be in pain anymore, that I promise."

"I . . . think that once [Gary] got his verdict and he was vindicated, and he knew there was money to take care of him, and that his wife was going to be secure, it wasn't too long after that that he died," Chad said. "I think he ceased fighting, because his fight was over, he had won . . . There was no reason he should have died that soon."

The last time David had talked to Gary, Gary had told him what to do with the money they got from the lawsuit.

David had a dream that Gary would be dead in thirty days.

"A baby bird in my window at work stared at me." David said. "It was Gary."

By the time David and Stacey got to hospital, Gary was on life support.

"The day was surreal," David said. "I got there with Stacey, and we talked to a doctor, who said, "Look, you have Option A, which is to let him keep going the way he's going; he will have a heart attack, and he will be suffering, and he will pass away. Option B is pull the plug, and let him go peacefully without any pain. What I said was, 'Doc, we're talking Option C, because I've heard Option A and Option B many times, and my brother has come back to us on at least seven, eight, nine, ten occasions where he's been gone and they said he's going to go, and he's come back. So I said, 'Where is Option C?' And he goes, 'There is no Option C.' And I said, 'Well, you better find one, because we're not listening to Option A or Option B. The only option is to let Gary go peacefully."

Carol, David, Stacey, Kenny, and Gary's sister, Barbara, gathered at Gary's bedside.

"Gary could hear us, even though he seemed unconscious," Carol said. "I'm sure of it."

Kenny played "Amazing Grace" on his cell phone.

When David had a private moment with Gary, he said, "I promise I'll make these people pay for what they did to you."

"I loved him," Barbara said. To Gary, she said, "I'm still here for you."

"The five years leading up to the day of pulling the plug was just, I mean I was, I felt, I don't know what I felt," David said. "I had to put on a brave face every day in front of my brother, but then I would leave crying every day in my car. I would come home, watch the TV with my family, but I'm not really watching TV, I'm just staring into space. And my mind is racing. Why is this happening, and you know, what's, why, you know, just why, why?"

He was so angry at the people who caused Gary to end up like this, he couldn't be coherent. Kenny stopped playing.

"I asked for Gary's last rites," Carol said. "And I asked for him to be baptized. Well, this preacher came in with a cotton swab. I put my hand on him."

"Is that holy water?" Carol asked.

No, said the preacher.

"My husband has accepted Jesus Christ," Carol said. "He deserves holy water, not just water out of the faucet. Could you please go find the bishop, and have him come up here and bless my husband?"

The bishop came and blessed him.

"Father, do you mind?" Carol asked.

No, he said.

Carol took a cotton swab and crossed his forehead.

"In the name of the Father, the Son, and the Holy Ghost, amen," Carol said. "Until we meet again."

She said the Lord's Prayer, which she had taught Gary. And which they frequently said together.

The doctors gave Gary medication to make him comfortable. The family formed a circle as the nurses started unhooking Gary from each machine that had been keeping him alive.

Carol watched his vitals.

"They were all dropping," Carol said. "It had gotten quiet."

Gary's heart was still going.

"We all said something to Gary about how much we loved him," Carol said.

"You'll be at peace now," Carol told Gary. "You don't have to worry. You'll be with Mom and Dad and Stevie. You're going to be reunited with them."

Carol was sure Gary heard them, because, she said, "hearing is the last thing to go."

David was undone.

"We were listening to bagpipe music," he said, "and I felt like I was having an out-of-body experience, like I was somewhere else, looking into the hospital room somehow. I was like, 'This isn't really happening, this can't be happening.' And then, and then it did happen. Now, we have to live with the aftermath every day, thinking about it, and seeing what we saw, and the quality of life that he had, or didn't have. You know, everything."

Carol thought she felt his heart beating. Two beats. As usual, Gary did everything in twos.

"He's still here," Carol said.

No one argued with her.

She thought Gary's agonized last breath was him fighting to stay alive.

"I just let her hold on to whatever she can hold on to," David said.

Somebody—Carol didn't know who—"took my hand and put it on Gary's heart. Somebody—he didn't know who—took David's hand and put it right next to mine. We felt the two strongest heartbeats my husband ever had, and then . . ."

Then: "I was watching the monitor," Carol said. "I knew he was gone."

Carol looked at the nurse and said, "He's passed away."

At 3:30, Gary was pronounced dead.

Barbara started crying.

"Barbara," Carol said, "please, just a couple more minutes. His heart has stopped, but he can still hear you, and I need him to hear that we love him, not tears."

Carol told Gary "I love you with all my heart, and I'm going to make sure you're okay. Everything still stays 50/50."

# 153

---

An RN told Carol she could only clean his face and hands.

"Is he your husband?" Carol asked.

No, he said. But I'm an RN.

"Can you change his wound vac?" Carol asked.

No, he said.

"I can," Carol said. "I think I can wash my husband."

The RN brought in water. It was cold.

"He may be cold but he wants warm water," Carol said. "I know my husband."

Carol's sister Linda knew Gary was having a Jewish funeral. She asked Carol if she also wanted a funeral in a church.

"This man changed his religion and took God, took Jesus into his life," Carol said, "And suffered for years. If anyone deserves to be in the front of that church, it's my husband. So yeah, I want him in that church."

"This part of Gary's life is closed," Carol said. "Now, we move on to a different life, which will never close."

Carol kissed Gary on the lips.

Willem had a necklace with a cross that came from the Holy Land. Her dad had kissed it. Jeanette kissed it. Carol kissed it. Gary kissed it. Willem held it as he died.

Gary would be buried with the necklace.

# 154

---

Around 5:30, Carol and David got back to Gary and Carol's house. Kimberly, Joel, and Nadilla joined them. They had said their good-byes in December. They watched movies from years earlier of Gary diving into the pool.

"Stacey, Kenny, and Kimberly took over," Carol said. "David and I were in really, really bad shape."

David was calling to Sol Levinson at the funeral home in Baltimore, "because," David explained, "they had taken care of my other brother and both my parents."

They planned to have a Jewish service in Baltimore in the next few days.

Linda took care of the arrangements for another funeral, a Christian service, in West Virginia.

"Gary really picked out the casket," Carol said, "not the exact one, but months earlier, online, Gary had pointed out which one he liked—a light blue coffin and he said he wanted something besides the white fabric on the top." Kimberly and Kenny found what Gary had wanted.

"He wanted a beach theme," Carol said.

"It was like steel," David said.

"It was different," Carol said, which was appropriate because "Gary was different."

The bank called Carol because of the number of large charges, and Carol explained that "my husband passed away, and this is what this money is for. For my husband. He is going to have the very best."

Gary didn't want to be buried.

"He wanted to be in an above-ground crypt next to my dad and my mom in Martinsburg, West Virginia," Carol said, "and he wanted me to be with him, and it was very important to Gary for Stacey to be buried next to David. And their parents and Stevie."

Carol knew how important it was for David and Stacey "to spend eternity next to each other. And he wanted us to spend eternity next to each other."

When Carol died, Gary's crypt could be opened and Carol could be slid in next to him.

"Our heads will be close to each other," Carol said.

The Martinsburg crypt was close to Jeanette's church, which kept Gary on their prayer list for years.

"Not a Sunday went by that the entire church was not praying for my husband," Carol said. "And when he would get bad during the week, I'd make a phone call, and it would start a chain and everyone would be praying for Gary that night."

At the funeral, Carol did not say good-bye. She never will.

# 155

After Gary's burial in the crypt, Carol fell apart.

She went to the end of Avalon Pier near their house in the Outer Banks where she and Gary had gone after Cleveland and threw flowers in the water.

"Right after Gary passed away, I had to go pick up some stuff at Wal-Mart," Carol said. "I went to the cashier."

Mrs. Stern, she said, How are you?

Carol started crying.

"Gary passed away," she told the cashier, who had been a nurse and had lost her job.

"I couldn't, I couldn't deal with Gary's death, so I just lay down," Carol said. "I kind of lost it. I lost it for a while. For months, and months, and months, I would have, and I still have them, but not as often as I used to, I have really bad nightmares about Gary. I've never told David just exactly what was going on in my nightmares, because it brought me to a really bad place, and I didn't want to do that to David."

"Carol," David said, "I'm sure I'm having the same nightmares."

"I would have nightmares that we would take the vac off," Carol said, "and Gary's intestines would start pouring out, and I would have to hold onto him and try and put them back in. The stool would be spewing out all over me, and Gary would be screaming. I was trying to catch his intestines before they hit the floor, and it was pouring out between, between my arms and trying to, and I kept just trying to, again, and again, and I just wanted to try and keep Gary alive. And then I would wake up, it was like that he was dead."

Carol started crying.

"Or I would wake up and realize that it was three o'clock," Carol said, "and it was time for me to change Gary's nightgown and his . . . his bed, because I always woke up at three o'clock in the morning to change him because he would have accidents, and I would wake up and he wasn't there. Or I would go to the refrigerator every day to pull out his TPN, even though I had just come from the bedroom crying because he wasn't there. And then

I would like, okay, get ahold of yourself, and then would get his TPN out of the refrigerator, and I would go and look and there's nothing there."

Carol couldn't stop sobbing as she told the story,

For eight years, Carol had been getting up between 2:00 and 4:00 to change Gary, to be sure he didn't have bedsores, to make sure he had dry clothes on. Without thinking, Carol got up and started doing those things for Gary.

"David and I had talked about how this wasn't going to be easy," telling Gary's story, "but I knew it was important to Gary, so I've got to get through it."

Carol dreamed about Gary after he got closed up in Cleveland and started getting sick again, about how Gary never threw up stomach contents again.

"He was throwing up stool," David said.

"That smell," Carol said. "I never, never, never let Gary see that it was offensive. There were times that Gary would have to wear a mask when I was changing him, because the smell was so bad, he couldn't stand it."

Carol never used a mask.

"Gary would beg me to put a mask on," Carol said, "and I would look at him, and I would hold his thigh, and or his forehead, and I would tell him that there is nothing that would ever come out of his body that would make me nauseous."

But in her nightmares Carol said, "all that stool would be still on me. The smell was stronger in my nightmares than I remember it being when I was actually changing him. Does that make sense? And I would have reactions, like he would see, it was like my worst nightmare: Gary seeing me in my dreams repelled by the stink."

After "we put Gary to rest," Carol added, "I wanted to die. I didn't want to be here anymore."

"Towards the end," David said, "Carol was dying with him, I mean, honestly, she was. She was run down to the point where she couldn't even put her head up.

"When we didn't have Gary anymore, everyone else was already used to the way it was, and we hid things from a lot of people. Not everybody saw the things that we did. There was just a handful of people who saw it. And so we didn't know how to react, because all of a sudden, all these things that we had built up in our heads for years, and years, and years, that we kept hidden, and never talked about, they were like circling all the time, and I think that's what really was bringing the nightmares out."

At times, Carol and David exchanged a look—as if they had a secret, which they did. The look was the same as the one they shared during the first invasive operation, when the doctors first took the bandage off.

"We knew not to go, 'Oh, my God,'" Carol said.

"We didn't want to scare Gary," David said. "We knew we had to hold back and keep it in, and we looked at each other and we're like, 'Oh, shit.' But we kept going, because we knew we were in a fight. We were in round six of fifteen rounds, and we had to keep fighting to stand up."

That was what they shared when they'd be in a group of people who were mourning.

"Everybody thought I was keeping Gary alive," Carol said—which meant to them somehow that Carol had failed.

"If I didn't have David . . .," Carol interrupted herself.

She couldn't find the words.

She explained that she and David "have to go through this so that we are able to help other people, and we are able to get Gary's story out." So other people suffering through something like this, including what they saw as the arrogance of the doctors, would know that others had gone through the same thing. They wanted to draw a map for other people.

# 156

"You want to know what the best kind of healthcare would have been?" Carol said. "The primary care physician should be allowed to consult whoever is in the ER. So that ER doctors know exactly what's going on. It would save millions."

"They won't share information," David said.

"Hospitals make it really hard for doctors," said Stacey, who, as a nurse, knew the medical business from the inside.

"Beside the bail bond business," David said, "I worked for my friend for the last ten years. Gamblers call us and pay for advice on who to wager on.

So, funny story, we have lawyers, doctors, judges, policemen who call us, to gamble."

One doctor would call while he was performing surgery.

"Doctors often have other things on their mind," David said.

About two weeks after Gary was buried, David found himself fighting the impulse to confront the doctors.

"I'm not sweeping this under the rug," David said. "In order for me to say to my brother, 'I'm going to make them pay,' this is the way that I can help others—instead of strangling the doctor."

Doctors can forget that they're holding lives in their hands and want to cover their asses and justify their decisions.

"And I finally confront one of the doctors," David said. "Their office is not far from mine. I went up there, and I said 'Is Dr. Heller in?' And they said, 'Are you a patient, sign in.' I said, 'I'm not a patient,' and she gave me a funny look, and she said to the guy next to her, 'Help this guy.' He goes, 'What's up?' I said, "Is Dr. Heller in?" And he goes, 'Who are you?' I said, 'David Stern, could you please let him know that I'm here to see him?' He calls in the back and says, 'Mr. Stern is here.' Dr. Heller wouldn't come out. He said, 'Tell him I'm not here.' So I said, 'Just thank Dr. Heller for misdiagnosing my fifty-two-year-old brother and putting him in his grave.' The entire place was in shock. Everyone turned around with their mouths open, all the employees, and the one or two patients. I never said the F word. 'Just tell him thank you.' And I walked out the door. But I want to look at the doctors in their eyes, and I want them to look at me in the eye. Because of what they took from me."

"David," Carol tried to calm David.

"What they took from us was just not fair," David said. He had no qualms about the effect of the trial on the doctors' careers and families. "Why shouldn't we take their Porsche, why shouldn't we take the steaks out of the refrigerator? Why shouldn't we take their home? They took a lot from us, something needs to be taken from them."

David also got a tattoo for Gary. His initials with a teardrop, "to remind us how much pain we have been in."

When everything was over but the grief, Carol called Southern Shore Pizza and ordered a lot of Gary pizzas.

"Anytime I get a big order like that," Boone, the pizza guy, said, "especially not in season, I ask . . . what was going on, is it like a party or something."

When Boone found out, he told his employees, because they always asked "How is Gary?"

The house was full. There were plenty of hungry mourners.

"Everybody was here because of Gary passing away," Carol said. "Everybody flew in."

Along with Gary pizzas, Carol got cream puffs with chocolate on the top, Gary's favorite.

After a long while, Carol said, "All Gary did was love me."

# Epilogue

---

We lived and learned, life threw curves
There was joy, there was hurt
Remember when

"Gary was and is my hero," Carol said a few years later. "I'm really missing him tonight."

The End